Praise fo
Healing the Pro

"Healing the Prostate *is every man's must-read. It's also a riveting book for women concerned about the health of the men in their lives too. Many men eventually need their prostate radiated, medicated, or operated on for various conditions, many of which could have been partially prevented. As an added perk, the science-based self-help tools in this healthy prostate plan will help keep many other organs healthy. I highly recommend this book!"*

— William Sears, M.D., author of *The Healthy Brain Book*

"*This is an easy-to-read, informative book covering the most recent research and treatments for the prostate and male genitourinary health. Dr. Stengler shares his clinical experience and case histories, and outlines practical diet and lifestyle recommendations, making the book relevant and useful for both the clinician and layperson. It is refreshing to see the inclusion of new perspectives for male health and a chapter dedicated to the bladder as a primary cause of male LUTS.*"

— Tracey Seipel, N.D., founder of Seipel Group, a nutraceutical company that pioneered the natural urological health category

"*Dr. Stengler has provided critical information that all men and their doctors need to know, especially men who are dealing with prostate or bladder disorders. The book is extremely well referenced, is easy to read, and gives valuable information about both conventional and integrative approaches to these very common problems.*"

— Frank Shallenberger, M.D., founder of The Nevada Center of Alternative and Anti-Aging Medicine

"I am a big fan of Dr. Mark Stengler because he produces results. His program for the prostate is 100% on target. Every man needs to read this book and follow his expert guidance to optimal health."

— Michael T. Murray, N.D., author of
The Longevity Matrix, DoctorMurray.com

"All men should become knowledgeable about prostate health because virtually all men will experience prostate health problems at some time in their lives. Unfortunately, many urologists recommend only traditional medical treatments for prostate health issues. Dr. Mark Stengler's book Healing the Prostate *provides men with a comprehensive overview of both conventional and holistic therapies for all issues related to prostate health. From erectile dysfunction and testosterone to BPH and prostate cancer therapies,* Healing the Prostate *is an educational book that I am happy to recommend to all men."*

— Ross Pelton, RPh, CCN,
The Natural Pharmacist, naturalpharmacist.net

"The numbers don't lie: 50 percent of all men will require treatment for symptoms of prostate enlargement, and 10 percent of men will develop prostate cancer in their lifetimes. Dr. Stengler has brought a commonsense approach to prostate health in his new book, Healing the Prostate. *Most of us would want to make meaningful changes in our daily routine if we thought it would decrease our risk of developing disease. Dr. Stengler gives a very concise and easily readable 'blueprint' on how to make those changes."*

— Carl Walker, M.D., board-certified urologist

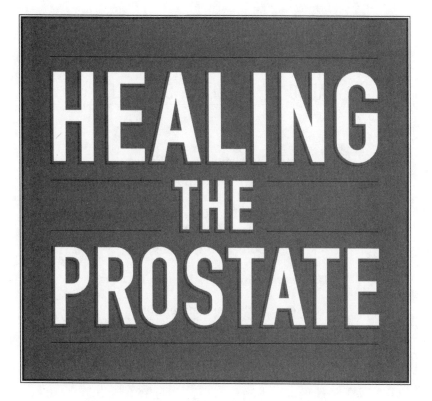

HEALING
THE
PROSTATE

ALSO BY DR. MARK STENGLER

Outside the Box Cancer Therapies,
with Dr. Paul Anderson*

Prescription for Drug Alternatives,
with James Balch, M.D.,
and Robin Young Balch, N.D.

The Natural Physician's Healing Therapies

Prescription for Natural Cures,
with James Balch, M.D.,
and Robin Young Balch, N.D.

*Available from Hay House
Please visit:

Hay House USA: www.hayhouse.com®
Hay House Australia: www.hayhouse.com.au
Hay House UK: www.hayhouse.co.uk
Hay House India: www.hayhouse.co.in

HEALING
THE
PROSTATE

THE BEST HOLISTIC METHODS TO TREAT THE PROSTATE AND OTHER COMMON MALE-RELATED CONDITIONS

DR. MARK STENGLER

HAY HOUSE, INC.
Carlsbad, California • New York City
London • Sydney • New Delhi

Published in the United States by: Hay House, Inc.: www.hayhouse
.com® • **Published in Australia by:** Hay House Australia Pty. Ltd.: www
.hayhouse.com.au • **Published in the United Kingdom by:** Hay House UK,
Ltd.: www.hayhouse.co.uk • **Published in India by:** Hay House Publishers
India: www.hayhouse.co.in

Cover design: Brad Foltz • *Interior design:* Julie Davison • *Interior illustrations:*
Courtesy of Shutterstock.com • *Indexer:* Joan Shapiro

Library of Congress Cataloging-in-Publication Data

Names: Stengler, Mark, 1969- author.
Title: Healing the prostate : the best holistic methods to treat the
  prostate and other common male-related conditions / Dr. Mark Stengler.
Description: 1st edition. | Carlsbad, California : Hay House, Inc., 2021.
Identifiers: LCCN 2020044135 | ISBN 9781401960346 (trade paperback) |
ISBN
  9781401960353 (ebook)
Subjects: LCSH: Prostate--Cancer--Alternative treatment.
Classification: LCC RC280.P7 S739 2021 | DDC 616.99/463--dc23
LC record available at https://lccn.loc.gov/2020044135

Tradepaper ISBN: 978-1-4019-6034-6
E-book ISBN: 978-1-4019-6035-3
Audiobook ISBN: 978-1-4019-6075-9

10 9 8 7 6 5 4 3 2 1
1st edition, January 2021

Printed in the United States of America

*To all the men looking for more
natural and holistic approaches
to preventing and treating
common male problems*

CONTENTS

FOREWORD

It is with great honor and pleasure that I introduce to you Dr. Mark Stengler's first prostate book. I've been waiting for this book since I met Mark about a decade ago at a natural medicine convention. I was starstruck when we met. After all, he is one of the most established writers in natural medicine and a highly regarded naturopathic physician.

At our first meeting, Mark had heard about my work in naturopathic urology, and he had a keen curiosity about the prostate and natural solutions for it. He had well-thought-out, detailed questions about the urinary system in men. At that time, I thought to myself, *It is only a matter of time before he writes a prostate book.*

Ten years later, we have this gem: *Healing the Prostate.* While most published books on prostate health lack expertise in natural solutions, or maybe are too dense for the common reader to understand, *Healing the Prostate* is grounded in scientific evidence while still being user-friendly and understandable for laymen. Based on my extensive clinical experience working with thousands of men with prostate issues of all kinds, I can assure you this book will help you prevent prostate problems or manage them with integrative therapies.

In this book, Mark takes you on a fascinating journey through the male anatomy, explaining how to keep it healthy with evidence-based, natural approaches. You'll come away with an appreciation for the prostate along with all the diseases that plague people who have one. When you find yourself getting into the weeds, it becomes evident that all those fine details regarding pathology, physiology, and so on are essential for understanding your options and guiding your course of action.

Healing the Prostate is comprehensively written, with solid advice and even recipes and resources to help you along your path toward vibrant health. It is an irreplaceable resource for laymen and physicians alike.

— **Dr. Geo Espinosa** is a naturopathic functional medicine doctor recognized as an authority in urology and men's health. He is faculty and holistic clinician in urology at New York University Langone Health and faculty for the Institute for Functional Medicine. As an avid researcher and writer, Dr. Geo has authored numerous scientific papers and books, including writing the best-selling prostate cancer book *Thrive, Don't Only Survive!* and co-editing *Integrative Sexual Health*. Dr. Geo is the chief medical officer and formulator at XY Wellness, LLC. He is writer and developer of the popular male health website DrGeo.com.

INTRODUCTION

The prostate gland is a wonderfully designed organ that serves many vital functions in the male reproductive system. However, for many men, dysfunction in this gland can cause this organ to feel like a curse.

In this book, you will discover how you (or the men in your life) can use diet, supplements, and lifestyle choices to support your prostate and overall health. You will also learn about the treatments available for a variety of male-related conditions, including benign prostatic hyperplasia (BPH), prostatitis, prostate cancer, hormonal imbalance, chronic pelvic pain syndrome, erectile dysfunction, low libido, and bladder and urinary tract issues.

WHY I WROTE THIS BOOK

All too often, patients complain that the medical system treats them like a number. At the Stengler Center for Integrative Medicine, all patients receive personalized care and health plans tailored to their unique needs and concerns. For optimal results, it's important that you understand what you can do at home to support your own health as well as all the professional treatments available to you— from the latest technological advances to the most powerful, time-tested traditions.

As a naturopathic medical doctor, I am well versed in both conventional and holistic medicine. In addition to the standard medical curriculum, which includes training in diagnosis, lab testing, pharmacology, and minor surgery, I have experience with bioidentical hormones, intravenous nutrient therapy, chelation therapy, ozone therapy, clinical nutrition, Chinese medicine, homeopathic medicine, botanical medicine, and even psychology and counseling. I also take research very seriously, constantly reviewing numerous medical resources for the latest treatments. I use my syndicated radio show, *Forever Young*, e-letters, television shows, and best-selling books to relay this knowledge to the hundreds of thousands of people who need it.

Healing the Prostate is designed to be a comprehensive yet user-friendly guidebook to the most effective therapies available today for various male-related conditions. Technical information is given in an easy-to-understand manner so that you can find and utilize the information that most interests you right away. (You can turn to the Endnotes if you'd like to dive deeper into the solid science backing my recommendations.)

The natural protocols for each of the men's health conditions are described with precise recommendations so that they can be discussed with your doctor and put into practice. It's important to communicate with your doctor regarding any protocols you wish to put into practice, especially for serious illnesses such as cancer. Proper monitoring is essential for the best health outcomes.

There are many factors involved in men's health, so consider this book just one resource as you do your research. For the most up-to-date health news, recommendations, and further resources to help you explore the topics in this book, please visit my website, www.markstengler.com. I hope the information contained within these pages empowers you to take charge of your health in a holistic way.

All my best,
Mark Stengler, N.M.D.

CHAPTER 1

HEALING THE PROSTATE— WHY EVERY MAN MUST TAKE ACTION

Why do we need to concern ourselves with the prostate? Odds are good that you, or someone you love, will be dealing with a prostate-related condition sometime during your life. Consider the following facts:

- One-third of men older than 50 years, and up to 90 percent of men by the time they've reached the age of 85, are affected by benign prostatic hyperplasia (BPH).[1]

- One in nine men will develop prostate cancer during their lifetimes.[2] Next to skin cancer, prostate cancer is the second most common cancer in American men.[3]

- Prostatitis is the most common urinary tract problem for men under the age of 50, and the third most common for men older than 50. Chronic prostatitis affects up to 15 percent of the American male population.[4]

- Many men with prostate problems also suffer from hormone deficiencies and imbalances. For example, low testosterone affects almost 40 percent of men aged 45 and older.[5] Hormone imbalances also play a role in a variety of men's health problems, including erectile dysfunction and low libido.

- Some men who are diagnosed with BPH and have urinary problems actually have bladder dysfunction.[6] In fact, approximately 3.4 million men in the United States have urinary incontinence. Some of these cases are related to an enlarged prostate, while others are bladder muscle problems.[7] This book will also address all bladder and lower urinary tract symptoms, not just the prostate-related ones, so that you can take a well-rounded approach to your health.

While the prostate can become diseased due to various factors, the good news is that your diet and lifestyle choices can reduce risk of these diseases and, in many cases, positively affect the treatment of these conditions if you already have them. Throughout this book, I discuss the tremendous benefit of scientifically proven nutritional supplements that set the stage for a healthy prostate and address other common men's health problems.

A QUICK GUIDE TO THE INTERESTING DESIGN OF THE PROSTATE

The prostate gland is an essential part of the male reproductive system. It is located within the pelvis and has two main lateral lobes (left and right) enclosed by a fibrous capsule. A normal prostate gland is about the shape and size of a walnut in younger men.[8] In older men, the prostate is larger and can range from the size of a Ping-Pong ball to that of a tennis ball.[9]

The prostate is located directly beneath the bladder and in front of the rectum. The upper portion of the prostate, known as the base, rests against the lower section (neck) of the bladder. The prostate's location below the bladder provides a type of structural support to prevent the bladder from dropping. It also creates space between the bladder and muscles and connective tissue in the area so that the vas deferens and seminal vesicles have room to connect to the urethra.[10] The prostate is composed of fibromuscular tissues that enclose many smaller glands and branching ducts.

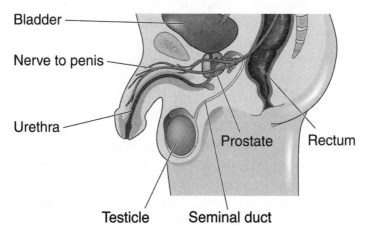

3

The prostate surrounds the urethra, the tube that drains urine from the bladder (and carries semen initially produced in the testicles) to the outside of the body. The prostate is encapsulated by tissues that include collagen, elastin, and high amounts of smooth muscle.[11] Muscles of the pelvic floor and their attaching ligaments are connected to the pubic bone in the front, to the coccyx bone in the back, and to your sitting bones (ischial tuberosity) and other structures that hold the prostate in place.

There are three main zones of the prostate:[12]

1. *Transition zone:* Where the urethra extends from the length of the prostate to the bladder neck. Benign prostatic hyperplasia occurs here and can lead to obstruction of the bladder outlet. Also, about 20 percent of prostate cancers occur in this region.

2. *Central zone:* The area surrounding the ejaculatory ducts. Cancers of the prostate are not common in this region.

3. *Peripheral zone:* The area covering the behind (posterior) and side (lateral) aspects of the prostate. This is the area where most prostate cancers are located and the region that is palpated by a doctor during a digital rectal examination (DRE). It is also the area that is most commonly affected by chronic prostatitis.

Some sources consider an area of the prostate known as the anterior fibromuscular stroma to be the fourth zone of the prostate.[13] This area is at the bottom of the prostate and the front (anterior) side. This region does not contain any glands, and prostate cancer is rare in this section.[14]

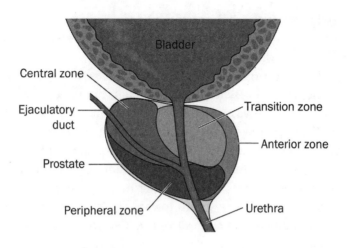

THE EXTENDED TEAM
OF THE PROSTATE

The prostate does not work in isolation. Instead, it is part of an extensive team of synergistic glands that participate in the production, maturation, and transport of sperm. This is how the prostate interacts with the other players.

Sperm are produced in each testicle, in structures known as the seminiferous tubules. The cells that manufacture the sperm are called Sertoli cells. Immature sperm are transported from the testes to long, coiled structures on the backside of each testicle known as epididymes. In the epididymes, sperm are stored and matured. When ejaculation occurs, sperm are expelled by contractive forces from each epididymis into a long, thick-walled tube known as the vas deferens (plural vasa deferentia), located in the pelvic cavity and behind the bladder. This pair of tubes carries mature sperm to the urethra to be released outside of the body during ejaculation.

The next organs involved in the process of ejaculation are the seminal vesicles, which are saclike pouches that are attached to the vasa deferentia near the base of the bladder. They produce a fluid containing fructose and citric acid, which provide the energy source for sperm to move, and prostaglandins, which make female cervical mucus receptive to sperm and cause uterine and fallopian tube contractions to move sperm toward the ovaries.[15] Most of the ejaculatory fluid comes from the seminal vesicles.

Next, the prostate gland secretes a thin, milky fluid that contains several compounds, including calcium, citrate ion, phosphate ion, a clotting enzyme, and an enzyme that breaks down blood clots (profibrinolysin).[16] When ejaculation occurs, smooth muscles inside the prostate gland contract simultaneously with the contractions of the vas deferens. This allows the slightly alkaline prostatic fluid to mix with the sperm, neutralizing the acidity of the fluid of the vas deferens, which is essential for fertilization of the female egg (ovum).[17] The alkalinizing effect of the prostatic fluid probably enhances the motility and fertility of sperm exposed to the acidic fluids such as the seminal vesicle fluids and vaginal secretions.[18] As a protective mechanism, the sphincter muscles of the prostate and bladder close the urethra so semen does not go upward into the bladder. Muscles contract during urination as well, closing the ducts to the prostate so urine cannot enter.

The bulbourethral glands, also known as Cowper's glands, are also involved, secreting fluid to lubricate the urethra for semen flow and to neutralize acidity from any urine residue in the urethra. The bulbourethral glands are located on the sides of the urethra, right below the prostate gland.

You may have heard of PSA, which stands for prostate-specific antigen. The PSA test is used by doctors to assess for prostate conditions such as benign prostate hyperplasia, prostatitis, and prostate cancer. While most men are concerned with PSA only as far as telling whether their levels are abnormal, it is important to note that PSA has a specific function. PSA is released along with prostatic fluid to liquefy semen after ejaculation, which allows sperm to travel more efficiently, and it has additional functions that are important for sperm fertility.[19] PSA also nourishes and protects sperm.

There are several hormones involved in sperm production.[20] These include testosterone, produced by specialized cells in the testis known as Leydig cells. Also, the front (anterior) portion of the pituitary gland, located at the base of the brain, secretes two hormones known as luteinizing hormone (LH) and follicle-stimulating hormone (FSH). LH stimulates the testis to produce testosterone, and FSH stimulates Sertoli cells of the testis to produce sperm. Both LH and FSH are released by the pituitary gland in response to signals from hormones produced by the hypothalamus section of the brain. Also, estrogens formed from testosterone are involved in stimulating sperm production.

Here is a summary of the production and transport of sperm:

- Hormonal messengers from the brain (hypothalamus to the pituitary gland) stimulate the testes to produce sperm and other hormones (testosterone, estrogen) that also stimulate sperm production.

- Sperm are produced in the seminiferous tubules of the testes by Sertoli cells.

- Immature sperm are transported to the epididymis, where they are stored and matured.

- With ejaculation, sperm are transported from the epididymis to the vas deferens.

- Seminal vesicles add fluid rich in nutrients that fuel sperm movement, such as fructose and citric acid, and prostaglandins that seem to aid fertilization.

- The prostate gland adds fluids and substances (including nutrients, enzymes, and PSA) that mix with the seminal vesicle fluid, nourish and protect sperm, and break down clotting, facilitating sperm movement and improving fertility potential.

- Bulbourethral glands secrete fluid that helps semen flow and neutralizes urine residue acidity.

You have read about all the glands, transport tubes, and substances involved in the production, storage, nourishment, and transport of semen, making it possible for an egg to be fertilized. This is a wonderful, elaborate design that allows for reproduction and life.

THE GENESIS OF
PROSTATE PROBLEMS

It's common sense that the environment to which cells are exposed has a significant influence on their health. The cells of the prostate are no different. Research continues to emerge demonstrating that modifications to exercise, weight, and diet can significantly affect common prostate problems. When these lifestyle factors are not appropriately controlled, it sets the stage for inflammation. Inflammation, especially chronic inflammation, is the body's response to irritation, and leads to unhealthy changes in cells and tissue.

Lower Urinary Tract Symptoms (LUTS)

Perhaps you experience waking up multiple times at night to urinate, frequent or urgent need to urinate, waiting for the urine flow to occur while standing at the toilet, a slow urinary stream, dribbling at the end of urination, and the inability to empty your bladder completely. These are all common symptoms of bladder inflammation and/or prostate enlargement. However, they can also be symptoms of a dysfunctional bladder and pelvic floor muscles. Due to the prostate being located below the bladder and encasing the urethra, men with prostate problems are prone to the aggravation of lower urinary tract symptoms (LUTS). I will describe therapies throughout this book that you can use to address these troublesome urinary symptoms.

Prostatitis

Prostatitis refers to infection or inflammation of the prostate gland, which may or may not involve an infectious agent (such as bacteria, viruses, or fungi). Prostatitis can be acute or chronic. If you have pelvic pain, difficulty or pain with urination, or pain with ejaculation, your doctor may order tests for prostatitis. Men with chronic prostatitis are often frustrated by the lack of effective treatment. Fortunately, there are effective natural options, which we'll discuss in Chapter 4.

Chronic Pelvic Pain Syndrome

Chronic pelvic pain syndrome (CPPS) may be a term that you are unfamiliar with. It is used to classify unexplained chronic pelvic pain in men without pus or bacteria visible on microscopic analysis of urine.[21] The type of pain varies depending on the cause. It can be sharp, dull, or cramp-like; it can be steady or intermittent. Holistic solutions for CPPS are also provided in Chapter 4.

Prostate Cancer

Prostate cancer is the second most frequent cancer diagnosis in men and the fifth leading cause of death worldwide.[22] Modern research has demonstrated that diet and lifestyle choices help reduce its likelihood and can be beneficial for men with nonaggressive forms that are following a watchful waiting (active surveillance) approach. Chapter 5 is dedicated to providing integrative cancer approaches for men with prostate cancer.

The Hormonal Connection

The prostate is a very hormone-sensitive gland. The prostate emerges in the fetus at 9 to 10 weeks gestation from the urogenital sinus, a channel from which the urinary and genital tracts open.[23] Importantly, during this embryological development, the prostate is dependent on a group of hormones known as androgens to stimulate growth.[24] This includes testosterone and, more importantly, its more potent metabolite known as dihydrotestosterone (DHT).[25] You will read more about the hormonal connections in the following chapters and especially Chapter 5.

DO INTEGRATIVE APPROACHES WORK?

Scientific literature, as well as my own experiences with patients at the Stengler Center for Integrative Medicine, provides overwhelming proof of the effectiveness of nutritional and integrative approaches for the prevention and treatment of common prostate conditions. Let me give you some examples of the major prostate conditions and how a holistic approach can be quite beneficial.

Benign Prostatic Hyperplasia

A 2019 review study analyzed the research on the influence of lifestyle modifications, nutrients, and herbal supplements on benign prostatic hyperplasia (BPH) symptoms. The researchers found that BPH symptoms can be improved through moderate exercise four to six times a week, a diet rich in vegetable protein and low in animal protein, and intake of vitamin D and zinc as well as supplements including saw palmetto, Cernilton, and *Pygeum africanum.*[26]

Prostatitis

A study published in the *British Journal of Urology* looked at the effects of a commercial rye pollen extract on 90 men with chronic prostatitis. These men were given one tablet, three times daily, for six months. Patients' symptoms were checked by laboratory tests and doctor evaluations after three and six months. Researchers found favorable results in 78 percent of the men: 36 percent were reported cured, and 42 percent improved.[27] This represents significant results for a condition that conventional medicine has difficulty treating.

Prostate Cancer

In 2005, noted holistic medical doctor and researcher Dean Ornish led a study on the effects of diet and lifestyle changes in men with prostate cancer. The study involved 93 men with early, low-grade prostate cancers who had declined conventional treatment such as radiation, surgery, or androgen deprivation therapy.[28] Patients were randomly assigned to one of two groups. One group was asked to make comprehensive lifestyle and diet changes. The other group was a control group, who did not make these lifestyle and diet changes.

At the end of the yearlong study, everyone in the lifestyle intervention group saw no increase in their prostate-specific antigen (PSA) levels nor progression of their prostate cancer based on magnetic resonance imaging (MRI). However, six of the control patients had to seek conventional treatment due to a worsening of their PSA or MRI results. PSA decreased 4 percent in the lifestyle and diet group but increased 6 percent in the control group. After two years, 2 of 43 patients in the lifestyle and diet change group underwent some type of conventional treatment, while 13 of the 49 control group patients had conventional treatment.

Mainstream studies like this demonstrate the potent effects of lifestyle and diet changes on prostate cancer progression.

Bladder Control

A unique study published in 2018 looked at the impact of an herbal combination known as Urox in the treatment of symptoms of an overactive bladder and urinary incontinence on men and women.[29] This herbal combination of concentrated extracts of *Crataeva nurvala* stem bark, *Equisetum arvense* stem, and *Lindera aggregata* root was found to improve urinary symptoms in 85 percent of users and had a 60 percent average reduction in urinary incontinence. This is quite the breakthrough in terms of natural products that exhibit significant benefits on urinary disorders.

HOLISTIC MEN'S HEALTH

The prostate gland should be viewed holistically, in terms of the whole body. Most men with prostate problems are also dealing with hormonal issues such as testosterone deficiency, estrogen elevation, and stress hormone imbalance. Moreover, tens of millions of American men have problems with low libido and erectile dysfunction. Since the body is interconnected in so many ways, especially when it comes to the influence of hormone balance on the prostate, this book covers these all-too-common male health problems. By bringing balance to the body's hormones, digestion, and musculoskeletal and urinary systems through better nutrition, detoxification, and stress reduction, one can achieve not only better prostate health but also better overall health.

CHAPTER 2

PROSTATE ENLARGEMENT (BPH) CAUSES AND SOLUTIONS

Harold, a 57-year-old entrepreneur, was sitting in my office as I was reviewing his health history when he stood up abruptly, saying, "It's ridiculous. I have to go all the time! Excuse me as I go to your restroom." As it turned out, Harold not only had frequent daytime urination problems but also had to get up to urinate three or four times every night, which disrupted his sleep and caused him to feel tired all the time. Fortunately, we were able to significantly improve his symptoms over the next two months through the use of a prostate-specific supplement combined with an herbal blend of bladder tonics.

◆ ◆ ◆

Benign prostatic hyperplasia (BPH) is an age-associated condition that involves enlargement of the prostate gland. This common condition affects approximately 50 percent of men between the ages of 51 and 60.[1] BPH becomes increasingly common as men age, with 90 percent of men at age 85 having this condition.[2] This condition is generally more severe and aggressive in African American men.[3]

The following urinary symptoms are indicative of BPH:[4]

- Incomplete emptying: bladder feels full even after voiding urine

- Increased frequency: need to urinate often, every hour or two

- Intermittency: the need to stop and start several times while urinating

- Urgency: sensation of needing to urinate right away

- Weak stream: a weak or feeble urinary stream

- Straining: need to push or strain to start urine flow

- Nocturia: the need to wake up at night to urinate more than two times

Men with severe cases of BPH end up with urinary retention, leading to hospitalization or surgery. Pharmaceuticals are conventional medicinal treatments for BPH, but they carry risks such as sexual dysfunction, breast enlargement, fatigue, decreased libido, and headaches.

CAUSES OF BPH

There are two main phases of prostate growth. The first phase is at puberty, when the prostate doubles in size. The second growth phase starts at around the age of 25 and continues through the rest of a man's life. It is during this second phase when BPH occurs.[5]

There is no single cause of BPH. Instead, there are likely several different causes, including genetic factors. However, one thing that researchers can agree on is that as men age, their hormone levels change, which affects prostate enlargement. Research has mainly focused on the hormones testosterone, dihydrotestosterone, progesterone, and estrogen.[6]

- *Testosterone:* The first thought for some people is that high testosterone is the likely culprit behind BPH. However, testosterone levels decrease as men age and their testosterone levels drop. We do not find BPH to be a problem with men in their late teens or early twenties, when testosterone levels are high. Moreover, castrated males, who have low testosterone levels, do not have issues with BPH.[7]

- *Dihydrotestosterone:* However, dihydrotestosterone (DHT), a metabolite of testosterone, *is* associated with BPH. Prostate gland tissue contains the enzyme 5-alpha-reductase, which converts testosterone into DHT. The hormone DHT binds to androgen receptors in the prostate and stimulates growth. (In the following section of this chapter, you will see that one of the major categories of drugs used to treat BPH inhibits 5-alpha-reductase so that less DHT is formed.)

   DHT stimulates prostate growth during fetal development in the womb. However, DHT continues to stimulate prostate growth later in life. Men with BPH have much higher levels of plasma DHT concentration compared to healthy men their age.[8] Furthermore, higher levels of DHT increases the enzymatic activity of 5-alpha-reductase, which may be related to BPH.[9]

Genetic variants in androgen receptors, known as polymorphisms, have been shown in some research to be related to BPH. These receptors, which are found in high concentrations in the prostate gland, influence the binding of testosterone and DHT as well as the regulation of genes that can affect the prostate.[10]

- *Estrogen:* Estrogen is another hormone that influences prostate growth. This hormone is a normal part of the male hormonal system, and most of it is produced in fat, brain, bone, and other tissues. The production of estrogen is primarily controlled by the enzyme known as aromatase, which converts the hormone androstenedione (synthesized by the testicles and adrenal glands) into the estrogen known as estradiol.

  Aromatase also converts testosterone from fat and muscle cells into estradiol. Increased activity of aromatase seems to be a causative factor in BPH.[11] Men tend to accumulate fat as they age, which leads to increased aromatase activity as well as decreased testosterone and elevated estrogen levels.[12]

  Age does not cause estrogen levels to decline the way it does testosterone.[13] The relative excess of estrogen in aging men compared to their testosterone (estrogen/androgen ratio) influences the later phases of BPH and prostate cancer.[14] There are two types of estrogen receptors inside prostate cells: ERα and ERβ. When estrogen binds to ERα, it stimulates prostate cell growth as well as prostate inflammation.[15] The binding of estrogen to ERβ, conversely, is antigrowth and anti-inflammatory, with the potential for anticancer effects.[16]

- *Progesterone:* Progesterone is also often thought of as a female hormone, but it also plays a role in men's health. It is produced in the adrenal glands and specialized testes cells known as Leydig cells, which also produce testosterone. The prostate gland has receptors for progesterone.[17]

There are other factors that may play a role in the formation of BPH, including elevated insulin levels (as seen with insulin resistance, e.g., prediabetes and diabetes), insulin-like growth factors, norepinephrine, and angiotensin II.[18] Other risk factors include a greater waist-to-hip ratio, obesity, and genetic predisposition.[19] There are also several nutritional imbalances associated with BPH, such as the high intake of animal protein, saturated fat, and cholesterol; high caloric intake; insufficient consumption of omega-3 fatty acids; and vitamin D deficiency.[20] We'll discuss the nutritional risks and solutions for BPH later in this chapter.

DIAGNOSING BPH

There are several different tests you might undergo to be diagnosed with BPH.

- *Questionnaire:* The first test you'll likely encounter is a questionnaire developed by the American Urological Association known as the BPH Symptom Score Index.[21] It has you rate your score based on urinary symptoms such as incomplete emptying, frequency, intermittency, urgency, weak stream, straining, and nocturia (getting up during the night to urinate), as well as your quality of life.[22]

- *Digital rectal exam (DRE):* The DRE is usually the next step in diagnosing BPH after a doctor reviews your urinary symptoms. This involves the doctor palpating the back wall of the prostate gland with a gloved finger coated with lubricant. The doctor is assessing the size of the prostate as well as the consistency of the tissue: whether it has a normal bogginess, has hard lumps, or is tender. (However, other tests may be done if your doctor is considering other prostate issues such as prostatitis or prostate cancer.)

- *Urine tests:* In addition, a urinalysis can be done, which would identify an infection, bleeding in the bladder or urinary tract, or assess urine flow. This is a noninvasive exam in which you will be asked to supply a urine sample in a cup. The sample would then be analyzed in a lab for white blood cells (indicating infection or inflammation) and red blood cells (indicating infection, inflammation, or more rarely benign or cancerous growths somewhere in the urinary tract).

- *The prostate-specific antigen (PSA) test:* This is a general screening blood test that measures PSA, which can be elevated with BPH, prostatitis, or prostate cancer.

Depending on your symptoms, your doctor may order other tests, including an ultrasound (to assess size and any structural abnormalities of the prostate), cystoscopy (to view the inside of the urethra or bladder using a scope with a camera), and an MRI.

CONVENTIONAL APPROACHES TO BPH

Conventional doctors, including family doctors and urologists, generally have little training in nutritional and holistic therapy, so their recommendations typically do not include nondrug and nonsurgical choices. The four main categories for conventional BPH treatments are as follows:[23]

Watchful Waiting/Active Surveillance

With this approach, one is closely monitored by a health professional but is not undergoing any therapies. The problem with this approach is that if symptoms do progress to a later stage, they may become more difficult to treat.

Medical Therapies

This approach includes the use or combination of BPH-specific medications, which are outlined in detail in the next section, "Pharmaceutical Approaches to BPH." These treatments can be helpful to reduce urinary symptoms, but there are numerous potential side effects. Instead, if possible, try the diet, lifestyle, and nutraceutical approaches in this book under an integrative doctor's guidance before resorting to medication.

Minimally Invasive Surgery

This category includes a number of different types of surgeries for men with moderate to severe BPH symptoms, such as the following:[24]

- *Prostatic urethral lift:* Small implants (stent-like devices) are placed in the obstructed urethra to push the enlarged prostate tissue out of the way of the urethra. One commonly used system is the FDA-approved UroLift.

- *Convective water vapor (steam) ablation:* Also known under the trade name Rezum, the treatment uses steam to destroy excess prostate tissue. A needle injected into the prostate transfers the steam used in the procedure.

- *Transurethral microwave thermotherapy:* This treatment uses microwaves to destroy excess prostate tissue. An antenna, transported inside a catheter, sends microwaves to the prostate.

- *Catheterization:* A catheter (a hollow, thin tube) is inserted through the urethra into the bladder to create a passageway for urine to drain. This is a temporary treatment for men who cannot empty their bladder rather than a therapy for BPH itself. It is often used while waiting for surgery or for medication to work.

A variety of side effects are possible from these minimally invasive surgeries, including urinary tract infection, burning with urination, more frequent urination, sudden urges to urinate, and blood in the urine. Less common side effects include retrograde ejaculation (semen flows backward to the bladder instead of forward) and erectile dysfunction.[25]

Surgery

You should not ignore BPH symptoms. If the prostate is so enlarged that it is obstructing the outflow of urine through the urethra, then it can result in complications such as a thickened, irritable bladder, which will affect bladder control; increased risk of bladder infection or bladder stones; and a backup pressure that can strain and damage the kidneys.[26] Situations that may warrant surgery include the following:[27]

- Inability to empty the bladder, which can result in kidney damage

- Inability to urinate after acute urinary retention (being unable to expel urine from the bladder)

- Incontinence as the result of an overfilled bladder or increased bladder sensitivity

- Bladder stones

- Residual urine (urine not expelled from the bladder) that is infected

- Recurring, severe blood in the urine

- Very poor quality of life due to severe symptoms

In order from least to most invasive, these are the types of surgery that can be performed for BPH:

- *Photoselective vaporization:* A cystoscope (a thin tube) is inserted through the urethra into the prostate so that a doctor can use a laser to destroy excess prostate tissue and stop bleeding.

- *Transurethral resection of the prostate (TURP):* A resectoscope (a thin instrument with a wire loop at the end) is inserted through the urethra to the prostate. An electrical current is passed through the wire to cut away excess prostate tissue and seal blood vessels. This is considered the conventional "gold standard" of BPH treatment, with marked improvement in approximately 93 percent of men with severe symptoms. However, the procedure causes impotence in approximately 5 to 10 percent of men and incontinence rates of 2 to 4 percent.[28]

- *Holmium laser enucleation of the prostate (HoLEP):* A laser is inserted with a special scope through the urethra to the prostate, where excess prostate tissue is destroyed.

- *Thulium laser enucleation of the prostate (ThuLEP):* Similar to the HoLEP, this procedure also uses a laser to destroy excess prostate tissue.

- *Transurethral electroevaporation of the prostate (TUVP):* An electrical current is transferred through a resectoscope to destroy prostate tissue and seal small blood vessels.

- *Transurethral water-jet ablation:* This procedure uses high-pressure water jets to destroy excess prostate tissue.

PHARMACEUTICAL APPROACHES TO BPH

Most conventional doctors prescribe BPH-specific medications for men who have more than mild LUTS and noncancerous, mildly enlarged prostate glands. Three main types of factors cause LUTS: *dynamic* (prostatic smooth muscle and bladder neck tone), *static* (enlargement of the prostate gland, causing mechanical obstruction), and *compensatory* (hypertrophy and irritability of the detrusor bladder muscle).[29] Most of the benefit of pharmaceutical therapy is from reducing dynamic and static factors.[30]

There are three main classes of drugs used to minimize LUTS and shrink or stop the increasing growth of the prostate: alpha-blockers, 5-alpha-reductase inhibitors, and phosphodiesterase-5 inhibitors.[31] Research has shown that combination therapy—combining two classes of medication—can be more effective in improving urinary flow and quality of life than use of a single drug.[32] Combinations may include finasteride and doxazosin, dutasteride and tamsulosin, and alpha-blockers and antimuscarinics.[33]

Alpha-Blockers

How they work: Alpha-blockers, in simple terms, block nerve impulses from stimulating certain receptors on prostate cells. They do so by inhibiting alpha-1a adrenergic receptors and blocking the effect of postganglionic synapses at the smooth muscle and exocrine glands.[34] This prevents prostate cell receptors from being stimulated to contract muscles of the bladder and prostate, resulting in relaxation of those muscles and allowing urine to flow more easily.

Options: Alpha-blocker options include tamsulosin, silodosin, terazosin, alfuzosin, phenoxybenzamine, and prazosin. Prazosin affects the dynamic factors of LUTS by relaxing the smooth muscles of the prostate and bladder neck. This action results in a widening of the urethral lumen and improved urinary flow.[35]

Effectiveness: Alpha-blockers are quite effective in reducing LUTS associated with BPH. Approximately 50 percent of users notice improvement between 48 hours and one week after initiating therapy. However, alpha-blockers do not reduce the prostate size or lessen the progression of BPH.[36]

A systematic review and meta-analysis evaluated whether newer BPH drugs (e.g., silodosin, darifenacin, fesoterodine, solifenacin, sildenafil) offered advantages over established treatments, primarily older alpha-blockers (e.g., tamsulosin, alfuzosin, doxazosin).[37] The researchers found that none of the new drugs or drug combinations used to treat LUTS caused by BPH were more effective compared with older alpha-blocker monotherapy.[38] Moreover, adverse events from the newer treatments or combinations were similar to or more significant than those from older alpha-blocker monotherapy when there was sufficient evidence to analyze.[39]

Side effects: Many side effects can be caused by alpha-blockers, including hypotension, heart fibrillation, floppy iris syndrome, abnormal ejaculation, erectile dysfunction, nasal congestion, dizziness, priapism, fatigue or weakness, extremity swelling, headache, nausea or upset stomach, and allergic reactions.[40]

5-Alpha-Reductase Inhibitors

How they work: The 5-alpha-reductase inhibitors (5-ARIs) treat BPH symptoms by inhibiting the conversion of testosterone to dihydrotestosterone (DHT) in the prostate. This leads to a decrease in prostate size because DHT may fuel prostate tissue growth.[41] For example, finasteride therapy for 36 months of treatment was shown to reduce prostate volume by 27 percent compared to baseline.[42]

Options: There are two main 5-ARIs: finasteride and dutasteride.

Effectiveness: These medications have been shown to reduce the progression of prostate growth and shrink the prostate, improving urine flow.[43] These drugs are more effective than alpha-blockers for men with larger prostate volumes (>40 mL) or PSA levels above 1.4 ng/mL.[44] However, these medications take longer to work (3 to 6 months)[45] than alpha-blockers and are only useful for moderately enlarged prostates.[46]

Side effects: Several side effects are possible with 5-ARIs, including impotence, allergic reactions, breast cancer, decreased libido, abnormal ejaculation, gynecomastia, and dizziness or lightheadedness.[47] The most common side effects are erectile dysfunction, decreased libido, decreased ejaculate, and decreased semen count, which can be irreversible.[48]

Previous research found these medications increased one's chances of acquiring high-risk prostate cancer. However, more recent research has shown that 5-ARIs reduce the risk of low-grade prostate cancer and cause no increased risk of death from high-risk prostate cancer.[49]

5-ARIs have a black box warning and are not approved for prostate cancer prevention.[50]

Phosphodiesterase-5 inhibitors

How they work: The phosphodiesterase-5 inhibitors (PDE5 inhibitors) work by inhibiting PDE5, which induces smooth relaxation in the lower urinary tract.[51] More specifically, PDE5 inhibitors reduce smooth muscle tone in the prostate, detrusor, and urethra via increased intracellular cyclic guanosine monophosphate.[52]

Options: The PDE5 inhibitor used for LUTS related to BPH is tadalafil.

Effectiveness: Tadalafil is less effective than alpha-blockers for improving urinary symptoms. However, since erectile dysfunction is a potential side effect of 5-ARIs, tadalafil can be used to counteract this problem and reduce LUTS.[53]

Side effects: There are several possible side effects with tadalafil. The most common include headache, myalgia, respiratory tract infection, nasopharyngitis, dyspepsia, flushing, back pain, nausea, and nasal congestion.[54] It is contraindicated for use with nitrates, a common medication for treating or preventing heart pain.[55] In addition, sudden hearing loss and erections lasting longer than four hours can occur.[56]

DOCTORS ARE USING HERBAL THERAPIES FOR BPH

The Urology Care Foundation demonstrates a drug-and-surgery-based system bias when they state on their website that "herbal therapy is not recommended by health-care providers."[57] This is a false statement, since holistic and integrative doctors by the tens of thousands in North America, Europe, and Asia recommend herbal therapy for the treatment of BPH. I know a holistic urologist whose clinic is within minutes of my office that recommends herbal therapies for BPH and other prostate and urinary problems. The same foundation's website also makes another blunder by stating, in regard to herbal treatment, "Several important studies show they don't work." What studies are they referring to? You will see later in this chapter that many studies back up the use of herbal therapy for BPH and urinary symptoms.

NATURAL APPROACHES

If you have been diagnosed with BPH, I would not advise waiting until you need pharmaceutical treatment or more invasive procedures. Instead, be proactive and follow the diet, lifestyle, and nutraceutical approaches outlined in this book. Work with your doctor to discover which holistic treatments will be helpful for you.

DIET

An increasing number of studies demonstrate a link between diet and BPH. The combination of obesity, reduced physical activity, and poor nutrition is known to alter the risk of symptomatic BPH and LUTS.[58] A recent review of the published literature on BPH and nutrition found some important patterns, as detailed below.[59]

The following are associated with higher risk of BPH:

- high protein intake from animal sources (but not vegetable sources)

- high intake of unsaturated fatty acids, which contribute to damaged cell membranes and increased 5-alpha-reductase activity (the conversion of testosterone to DHT, which may fuel prostate growth)

- high intake of foods rich in saturated fat and high in cholesterol, which can promote inflammation

- high caloric intake, which can increase abdominal obesity and sympathetic nervous system activity

- intake of high-glycemic foods such as bread, pasta, and rice that are associated with increased serum insulin and insulin-like growth factor, which may stimulate BPH (no association was found with the intake of high-glycemic fruit)

- high coffee intake, which stimulates the adrenergic nervous system and smooth muscles of the prostate, which can worsen BPH symptoms

The following are associated with lower risk or improved symptoms of BPH:

- omega-3 fatty acids (found in foods such as cold-water fish, vegetables, ground flaxseed, and flaxseed oil), which reduce inflammatory compounds that create inflammation related to BPH

- lignans (found in whole flaxseeds), which promote estrogen removal and may protect against BPH

- garlic extracts, regular consumption of which has led to improvements in disease parameters in BPH patients

- phenols (found in cranberries and other dark-colored grapes and berries), which may help with LUTS

Studies are mixed on the effect of alcohol on BPH. See Chapter 8 for more detailed dietary information and the Appendix for meal-planning recommendations.

EXERCISE

There are several studies suggesting that exercise may protect against BPH and LUTS by reducing body size, decreasing sympathetic nervous system activity, and reducing levels of inflammation. In one review of studies, physical activity was strongly associated with reduced nocturia (nighttime urination). Men who are active for one hour or more per week are 34 percent less likely to report severe nocturia compared to men who reported no physical activity.[60]

Recommendation: A minimum of 30 minutes (preferably 60 minutes) of moderate daily exercise

SUPPLEMENTS

As an integrative doctor, I recognize that some men with BPH do exceptionally well using solely natural approaches, while others require conventional methods as well. Approximately 40 percent of American men who choose nonsurgical treatment of BPH use herbal supplements alone or with other medications.[61] After reading through the supplements recommended here, review the proper course of action for you with your doctor. Note that the recommended doses here are specifically for the prevention and treatment of BPH, not for general health purposes.

Beta-Sitosterol

Beta-sitosterol is one of several plant sterols. It is found in most plants, with higher amounts in rice bran, wheat germ, soybeans, corn oil, peanuts, avocados, pumpkin seeds, cashew fruit, saw palmetto, and *Pygeum africanum*.[62] Sterols are steroids produced by plants and are structurally and functionally related to cholesterol. Beta-sitosterol is the most abundant plant sterol consumed by humans.[63]

Beta-sitosterol inhibits 5-alpha-reductase enzyme and has anti-inflammatory properties. Research has demonstrated that beta-sitosterol supplementation improves BPH symptoms such as urinary symptom scores and flow measures better than placebo.[64] In a study of 200 men with BPH, the men were given either 20 mg of beta-sitosterol three times daily or a placebo. Those taking beta-sitosterol had significant improvements in urinary flow, while the placebo group did not have changes.[65] Another study demonstrated that 177 men with BPH supplemented with 130 mg of beta-sitosterol daily had significant improvements compared to placebo in terms of urinary parameters and quality-of-life score.[66] However, beta-sitosterol has not been shown to reduce the size of the prostate gland.[67]

Recommendation: 60 to 130 mg daily

Safety: Beta-sitosterol has an excellent safety rating.

Rye Pollen Extract

Rye pollen extract (also known as ryegrass flower pollen, ryegrass, or flower pollen extract) has been an herbal treatment in Europe for many decades. There are several studies demonstrating its effectiveness in reducing the symptoms of BPH.

Recent research has shown that Cernitin, a well-researched type of rye pollen extract, regulates inflammatory chemicals known as cytokines in prostate cells and decreases androgen receptor levels.[68] In a 12-week study of men with BPH supplementing Cernitin at a dosage of 126 mg three times daily, overall clinical effectiveness was 85 percent.[69] Symptoms that were significantly improved included urgency, dysuria (pain or difficulty with urinating), nocturia, incomplete emptying, prolonged voiding, delayed voiding, intermittency, and dribbling at the end of urination. In the same study, 28 out of 79 men treated for more than one year had a decrease in mean prostate volume.

A study published in the journal *International Urology and Nephrology* examined the effectiveness of Cernitin in combination with other nutraceuticals, including saw palmetto, beta-sitosterol, and vitamin E.[70] The study involved 144 men enrolled in three different urological practices. When compared to placebo, the combination product significantly reduced nocturia and overall BPH symptoms per the American Urological Association Symptom Index score, with no significant adverse effects.

Recommendation: 126 mg three times daily, up to 500 mg daily

Safety: Side effects are uncommon but may include digestive upset.

Saw Palmetto

Saw palmetto berries and extracts are a popular herbal therapy for the treatment of BPH in North America and Europe. This plant has a long history of use by Native Americans for the treatment of prostate and urinary problems, and this practice was later adopted by American settlers and Europeans. Around half of German urologists prefer to prescribe plant extracts such as saw palmetto rather than pharmaceuticals for BPH.[71] Several studies have proven the effectiveness of saw palmetto in improving the symptoms of BPH, mainly focusing on the extract form containing a standardized fat-soluble (liposterolic) product containing 85 to 95 percent fatty acid and sterols.

Saw palmetto has multiple mechanisms that are likely responsible for reducing BPH symptoms. It has antiestrogenic effects and inhibits the conversion of testosterone into DHT in prostate tissue and intracellular binding to receptors in the prostate.[72]

As with other herbal therapies, saw palmetto works best for mild to moderate symptoms in the early stages of BPH. About 90 percent of men notice an improvement in mild to moderate urinary symptoms of BPH within the first four to six weeks of starting supplementation with 320 mg per day of a liposterolic extract.[73]

A 2018 paper conducted a saw palmetto systematic review and meta-analysis of randomized controlled trials and observational studies of men with BPH. The data included a total of 27 studies. Researchers found that saw palmetto extract reduced nocturia and improved maximum urinary flow compared to placebo. Furthermore, saw palmetto extract had a similar benefit to those of the drug tamsulosin and a 5-alpha-reductase inhibitor in relieving LUTS. There was no negative effect on sexual function or PSA levels. There was a slight decrease in prostate size (volume). The authors concluded that saw palmetto extract "appears to be an efficacious and well-tolerated therapeutic option for the long-term medical treatment of LUTS/BPH."[74]

In another review involving 21 randomized trials lasting between 4 and 48 weeks, when compared with a placebo, saw palmetto improved urinary symptom scores, symptoms, and flow measures.[75] Also, saw palmetto produced similar improvements in urinary symptom scores compared to the drug finasteride and had less adverse events than finasteride.

Some older studies have questioned the effectiveness of saw palmetto for relieving BPH symptoms.[76] Why would so many previous studies demonstrate significant benefits then? My colleagues Dr. Geo Espinosa and Dr. Michael

Murray have insight into this discrepancy, and the answer focuses on how severe the BPH is when men first start supplementing saw palmetto. In *Textbook of Natural Medicine,* they note:

> The chance of clinical success with any of the botanical treatments of BPH appears to be determined by the degree of obstruction, as indicated by the residual urine content. For levels less than 50 mL, the results are usually excellent. For levels between 50 and 100 mL, the results are usually quite good. With residual urine levels between 100 and 150 mL, it will be tougher to produce significant improvements in the customary 4- to 6-week period. If the residual urine content is greater than 150 mL, saw palmetto extract and other botanical medicines alone are unlikely to produce any significant improvement.[77]

Another likely reason why some studies have not found saw palmetto to be effective has to do with the composition of the extracts studied, which affects their biological activity. One negative review noted this weakness in their saw palmetto analysis: "It is not possible to be absolutely certain that these findings apply to all saw palmetto extract preparations, given the unknown active ingredients and unknown mechanism of action."[78]

Several positive studies of saw palmetto for reducing LUTS from BPH have been done using extraction techniques other than hexane and supercritical CO_2 extracts. Other extraction techniques would not yield the same type of active constituents. Published meta-analyses often used a broader range of products with different compositions of various substances based on different extraction techniques.[79]

A recent article published in *Food Science and Biotechnology* found the efficacy of saw palmetto extract depends on the type of standardized formula.[80] In other words, how the product is manufactured and extracted, and the resulting concentration of bioactive constituents, seems to be very important. The authors noted that free fatty acids at a level of greater than 80 percent provided more consistent results. Also, free fatty acids (lauric acid) were effective in inhibiting 5-alpha reductase, and beta-sitosterol reduced prostatic inflammation. Proper standardization of multiple bioactive components of saw palmetto extract seems necessary for good and consistent outcomes in the alleviation of BPH symptoms.

Published studies show that the combination of saw palmetto and stinging nettle root extract is effective in reducing LUTS associated with BPH.[81] I have written more about this in the following section on nettle root.

Recommendation: 320 mg daily of a liposterolic extract that is standardized to 80 percent or higher fatty acids

Safety: A review of studies on saw palmetto for the treatment of BPH found that it was well tolerated and not associated with serious adverse events. Also, there was no evidence of drug interactions.[82]

Pygeum africanum

Pygeum africanum, also known as *Prunus africana*, has a history of use in Africa for urinary disorders.[83] The active components of *Pygeum africanum* appear to be ferulic acid esters, which lower cholesterol within the prostate and reduce metabolites that contribute to prostate growth.[84] Furthermore, *Pygeum africanum* contains sterols that reduce inflammatory compounds that cause inflammation; they also reduce testosterone accumulation within the prostate.[85]

A study published in *The Prostate* found that *Pygeum africanum* has antiproliferative and apoptotic (causing natural cell death) effects on certain types of tissue (fibroblasts and myofibroblasts) without affecting the smooth muscle cells of the prostate gland.[86] *Pygeum* appears to have beneficial, LUTS-reducing effects on both prostate and bladder tissue.[87]

A review of 18 randomized controlled trials involving 1,562 men and ranging between 30 and 122 days was positive. Compared to placebo, *Pygeum africanum* "provided a moderately large improvement in the combined outcome of urologic symptoms and flow measures." Those supplementing *Pygeum africanum* were more than twice as likely to report an improvement in overall symptoms, nocturia was reduced by 19 percent, residual urine volume decreased by 24 percent, and peak urine flow increased by 23 percent. Side effects were mild and comparable to placebo.[88]

A different study published in the journal *Urology* involved 209 patients with BPH who were given either 50 mg twice a day or 100 mg once daily for two months, and then an open phase where 174 patients received 100 mg daily. The results were similar in both phases with regard to effectiveness and safety. After 12 months of treatment, there was even further improvement.[89]

A review authored by urologists of the evidence for the treatment of BPH with *Pygeum* concluded that its long history of use, along with strong enough published data, makes it "a useful drug for the urologist."[90]

Recommendation: 100 to 200 mg daily of a standardized extract (usually 14 percent triterpenes)

Safety: *Pygeum africanum* has no significant side effects but may cause gastrointestinal upset.[91]

Nettle Root

Research has shown nettle root, more specifically stinging nettle (*Urtica dioica*), to be effective in treating BPH. Stinging nettle root has a traditional use in Europe for the treatment of urinary tract infections.

The mechanisms for this effectiveness appear to be multifactorial but research has not isolated them definitively, including the inhibition of sex hormone–binding globulin binding to prostate receptors, reduced conversion of testosterone into estrogens by reducing aromatase activity, and anti-inflammatory effects on prostate tissue.[92]

A double-blind, placebo-controlled, randomized study compared nettles with placebo in 620 patients. During the six-month trial, more of those receiving nettles (81 percent) reported improved LUTS compared with patients in the placebo group (16 percent). Also, those taking nettles had a reduction in postvoid residual urine volume (amount of urine left in the bladder after urination) from an initial value of 73 to a final value of 36. In contrast, those on placebo saw no appreciable change. There was also a modest decrease in prostate size as measured by ultrasound in the nettles group but none in the placebo group. No side effects were found in either group. At the end of the trial, the placebo group began taking nettles, and an 18-month followup found improvement only in those who continued with the therapy. [93]

In another double-blind clinical trial, 100 men with BPH between the ages of 40 and 80 were given nettles (300 mg twice daily) or a placebo for two months. Those taking nettles had significant improvements in urinary symptoms, and those on placebo had no change. The authors noted, "Nettle is recommended to be used more in treatment of BPH patients, given its beneficial effects in reducing BPH patients' symptoms and its safety in terms of its side effects and its being better accepted on the side of patients."[94]

The combination of nettle root and saw palmetto is popular in nutraceutical formulas. In one double-blind clinical trial, the combination of 160 mg of saw palmetto and 120 mg of nettle root was evaluated in 257 elderly men with moderate or severe LUTS caused by BPH.[95] The men were treated with this combination or a placebo for 24 weeks, which was followed by a 24-week control period, then a 48-week follow-up period in which all men received the herbal combination. Assessment at week 96 revealed that the International Prostate Symptom Score (IPSS) was reduced by 53 percent, peak and average urinary flow increased by 19 percent, and residual urine volume decreased by 44 percent in the treatment group. The remedy was very well tolerated. Additional published studies, including one published in the *World Journal of Urology*, have shown benefit for treating LUTS related to BPH with this combination.[96]

Recommendation: 120 to 600 mg daily

Safety: The safety rating is very good for nettle root.

Pine Bark Extract

Pycnogenol is a patented form of French maritime pine bark extract. It contains a number of plant compounds, including procyanidins, bioflavonoids, and phenolic acids, that have a number of therapeutic effects such as reducing inflammation. There have been approximately 450 scientific publications and 160 clinical trials on this natural substance, a lot more than the vast majority of drugs can claim.

An eight-week study published in 2018 and involving 75 men compared the standard management protocol (routine exercise, hydration, and a low-sugar and low-salt diet), the same protocol plus 150 mg Pycnogenol daily, and the standard pharmacological management of finasteride and dutasteride. After eight weeks, the participants were evaluated with ultrasound to determine residual urinary volume in the bladder as well as prostate size. Results of the study found significant improvement in BPH symptoms with the use of Pycnogenol as compared to both control groups, and with no adverse effects:[97]

- Bladder emptying improved by 42 percent in the treatment group as compared to 9 percent in the control.

- Frequency of urination was reduced by 37 percent in the treatment group as compared to 12 percent in the control.

- Nocturia frequency was reduced by 31 percent in the treatment group as compared to 18 percent in the control.

- Improvement of weak flow improved by 24 percent in the treatment group as compared to 9 percent in the control.

Recommendation: 150 mg Pycnogenol daily
Safety: If you are on anticoagulant therapy, check with your doctor before using this supplement.

Zinc

The mineral zinc is found in high concentrations in the prostate.[98] It plays a vital role as a constituent of prostatic fluid as well as influencing healthy prostate development and functioning. High-zinc food sources include shellfish, beef and other red meats, nuts, and legumes. The recommended daily allowance (RDA) for adult men is 11 mg, or 8 mg for women.

The scientific evidence for zinc supplementation is relatively weak compared to the other natural substances reviewed in this chapter. However, a study published in the *American Journal of Epidemiology* found that higher zinc intake (>23 mg) was associated with a lower risk of BPH.[99] Also, another study found a significant decrease in prostate zinc levels in men with BPH as compared to normal prostate tissue.[100]

Recommendation: For long-term usage, 25 to 30 mg daily, with meals

Safety: At normal doses, zinc supplementation is quite safe. Mild digestive upset can occur with doses of 50 mg and higher.[101] Zinc supplementation of more than 50 mg a day that continues for several weeks should be accompanied by copper supplementation to prevent copper deficiency.[102]

Vitamin D

Prostate tissue has vitamin D receptors, which influence prostate tissue metabolism and the ability to control inflammation. Research suggests that men over the age of 50 with LUTS have lower levels of vitamin D than men without.[103] Another study published in *Urology* found that there is a relationship between vitamin D deficiency and urinary symptoms associated with prostate growth, as found with BPH. The same authors noted that low vitamin D promotes cell proliferation and apoptosis in healthy prostate cells.[104]

Vitamin D deficiency is common in American men and is associated with moderate to severe urinary incontinence and at least one lower urinary tract symptom.[105]

Recommendation: 2000 to 5000 IU daily, with a meal. However, dosing is best based on serum vitamin D (25-hydroxyvitamin D) levels. A level of 50 ng/mL is a decent serum vitamin D level.

Safety: Vitamin D is considered to be a safe supplement at regular dosages. Levels can be monitored with blood testing.

Fatty Acids

Fatty acids play a role in cellular health in tissues of the body. Essential fatty acids (EFAs) are required in the diet since the body cannot manufacture them. EFAs are precursors to a group of chemical messengers known as prostaglandins.

Research going back to 1999 demonstrates that serum levels of omega-3 fatty acids are significantly decreased in men with BPH.[106] There is not a lot of research in terms of omega-3 fatty acid supplementation and the treatment of BPH. However, in one study of 100 men who had LUTS and BPH, the men were randomized to receive either the BPH drugs tamsulosin and finasteride or the same drugs along with omega-3 fatty acids three times a day. The group receiving omega-3 fatty acids showed greater improvement in urinary symptoms and more improvement in prostate volume at month six.[107]

Recommendation: 1000 mg daily of EPA and DHA

Safety: Omega-3 fatty acids are safe. Check with your doctor before supplementing if on blood-thinning or anti-coagulant medications.

OTHER INTEGRATIVE TREATMENTS: ACUPUNCTURE

Acupuncture has been demonstrated to be effective in treating BPH. A systematic review showed that acupuncture caused statistically significant changes in the short-term follow-up end points of patients with moderate to severe BPH.[108] A separate review of studies involving 661 men found statistically significant changes in favor of acupuncture for men with moderate to severe BPH.

Recommendation: Consult with a licensed acupuncturist for proper acupuncture therapy.[109]

THE BLADDER FACTOR FOR BPH AND URINARY CONTROL

Sean, a 66-year-old male, came to my clinic for long-standing prostate problems. He explained that his BPH was causing him to get up six times a night, leading to fatigue and poor concentration the next day. He also had frequent urination during the day. When I asked him what he had been taking for his BPH, he held up a bag of different prostate formulas. Unfortunately, they were not making much difference for him. I told Sean to continue with one supplement that I felt had good value, but to also add a bladder formula to his protocol. This particular formula, Urox, contains a blend of three herbs that have been shown in published research to reduce urinary symptoms. When Sean followed up three months later, he was delighted with the results. He told me how his daytime urination frequency had improved, and more impressive was that his nighttime urination frequency now averaged one to two times a night.

◆ ◆ ◆

Men have been battling urinary problems for centuries. Ancient documents such as the Indian surgical text Sushruta Samhita, dated around 1000 B.C., describe the use of gold, silver, iron, or wood smeared with liquid butter (ghee) as a type of catheter to relieve urinary retention.[1] It was also recommended to drink wine before this procedure to reduce pain![2]

Some of the most problematic symptoms for men with BPH are urinary symptoms, for which treatments for BPH are often helpful. Fortunately, the holistic therapies discussed in Chapters 2 and 3, especially the simple-to-use and nontoxic herbal therapies I address, are especially effective and convenient. However, for many men with BPH, their bladder is the main source of their urination problem; BPH is in fact the secondary problem. The medical literature acknowledges that some men with urinary problems who are diagnosed with BPH actually have bladder dysfunction instead.[3]

This is why, in recent years, I have seen a much higher response rate in men with BPH and urinary symptoms when there is accompanying holistic treatment for the bladder and urinary system. This approach has been a game changer in terms of helping men with their urinary problems. Following the treatments for urinary control in this chapter will help men with BPH, bladder problems, or a combination of both issues with their lower urinary tract symptoms (LUTS), including the following:[4]

- *Storage symptoms:* increased bladder sensation, frequency, urgency, urge incontinence, nocturia

- *Emptying symptoms:* hesitancy, dysuria, intermittency, a small amount of urine, dribbling at the end of urination, and sensation urine still needs to be voided

- *Painful symptoms:* pelvic pain, perineal pain, and urethral pain

THE CAUSES OF LUTS

There are several causes of LUTS. For example, many men have bladder problems that cause storage and emptying symptoms.[5] The effect on symptoms is compounded when BPH is involved; severe BPH results in obstruction of the bladder outlet, because the prostate is located at the bottom of the bladder. This is known as bladder outlet obstruction (BOO).[6]

Many men, especially older men, have overlapping problems (their prostate enlargement obstructing the bladder) and direct bladder problems. A lot of men have an overactive bladder (OAB) due to bladder dysfunction, such as an overactive or impaired bladder muscle (detrusor muscle).[7] One study found that the incidence of OAB in men was more than double what was previously reported.[8]

A doctor assesses the severity of LUTS through observing a man's symptoms as well as having the patient complete questionnaires. Questions often address the following:[9]

- symptom frequency and severity
- variation between nighttime and daytime symptoms
- precipitating or relieving factors
- prior treatments and their success
- coping measures used by the patients to improve their symptoms
- the impact of the symptoms on quality of life and social function

The International Continence Society recommends keeping a three-day bladder diary.[10] Patients record the time they wake up and go to bed, fluid intake, food intake (while assessing the water amount in foods), the volume of urine passed each time they urinate, each episode of incontinence, and use of incontinence pads.

In addition to a physical exam and urine analysis, your doctor may also order imaging studies of the urinary tract (such as ultrasound or CT scan), urodynamic studies (such as urine flow and pressure measurements), and, less often, a urinary tract endoscopy (camera view inside the urinary tract).

OVERACTIVE BLADDER (OAB)

OAB refers to a group of urinary symptoms that affects up to 30 percent of men in the United States.[11] The most common symptom is a sudden, uncontrolled need or urge to urinate.[12] For some men, OAB causes leakage of urine. An additional symptom is the need to urinate many times during the day or night. OAB is different from incontinence, where there is a leakage of urine.

The muscle that surrounds the bladder is known as the detrusor. When the bladder is full of urine, stretch receptors in the bladder wall trigger a nervous system reflex that causes the detrusor muscle to contract. This forces the urine toward the urethra to be expelled. Your bladder has an internal urethral sphincter that relaxes for urine to pass out. This internal sphincter is under the involuntary control of your nervous system. There is also an external urethral sphincter that you have mostly voluntary control over. The external urethral sphincter must relax for urine to pass into the urethra to flow outside the body. Approximately 69 percent of men with OAB have an overactive detrusor muscle.[13]

Risk factors for OAB include the following:[14]

- neurological disorders and diseases or injuries of the brain or spinal cord (e.g., stroke, multiple sclerosis)
- hormone changes
- pelvic muscle weakness or spasms
- urinary tract infections
- advanced age
- diabetes
- BPH
- prostate or pelvic surgery
- radiation therapy to the pelvis
- obesity

Conventional Approaches to OAB

There are several conventional medical approaches to OAB that include behavioral therapy. Habit modifications that you may be asked to do include the following:

- preplanning bathroom visits
- changing drinking habits
- eating different foods
- weight loss (for those who are overweight or obese)

- reducing fluid intake
- decreasing or eliminating caffeine

The first stage of treatment may also include pelvic floor exercises, such as these:

- Kegel exercises, which improve pelvic muscle and pelvic floor muscle tone
- biofeedback therapy, where one learns how to control one's pelvic muscles and improve bladder control through nervous system control
- direct physical therapy such as pelvic floor electrical stimulation

If these types of behavioral therapy are not effective, then the use of drugs or surgery may be needed. There are several different medicines that doctors may prescribe to relax the bladder muscle:

- *Anticholinergics:* As the name implies, this category of drugs has the action of inhibiting the neurotransmitter acetylcholine from binding to specific receptors (muscarinic) in the bladder detrusor muscles, which decreases involuntary bladder contractions. Examples of these drugs include tolterodine (Detrol), oxybutynin (Gelnique), trospium, darifenacin (Enablex), solifenacin (VESIcare), and fesoterodine (Toviaz).

  Common side effects of these medications include dry mouth, constipation, facial flushing, and blurry vision, as well as confusion in the elderly.[15]

- *Beta-3 adrenergic agonists:* This class of drugs includes the drug mirabegron (Myrbetriq) that inhibits nerve transmission to the detrusor muscle, which causes a relaxation of the bladder wall. The most common side effects of this medication include headache, high blood pressure, constipation, dizziness, diarrhea, back pain, dry mouth, joint pressure, and common cold symptoms.[16]

- *Tricyclic antidepressants:* The antidepressants imipramine and doxepin are sometimes used for OAB, working to decrease bladder contractility. Side effects may include fatigue, dry mouth, weakness, constipation, blurred vision, digestive upset, and confusion.[17]

A study published in *JAMA Internal Medicine* found that people 65 and older using anticholinergic medications had a higher risk of dementia. This class of drugs is known to have the risk of impaired cognition, including working memory, attention, and psychomotor speed. Also, observational studies have found that the discontinuation of these drugs may not reverse cognitive problems, including mild cognitive impairment or dementia.[18]

Botox may be injected therapeutically into the detrusor muscle of men who do not respond to drug therapy. Botox prevents the release of acetylcholine so that there is a reduction in bladder muscle contractions. The effects of these injections are temporary, and they may need to be repeated every four to six months. Potential side effects include urinary retention (being unable to urinate), which requires treatment with catheterization until the drug wears off.[19]

URINARY INCONTINENCE

Urinary incontinence, another component of LUTS, refers to the accidental leakage of urine.[20] Up to one-third of men suffer from urinary incontinence.[21] There are four main types:[22]

- *Stress incontinence:* urine leakage from abdominal and bladder pressure created from laughing, sneezing, coughing, or other stressors. (Can be a side effect of prostate surgery or radiation therapy.)

- *Urge incontinence:* the involuntary loss of urine that is preceded by urgency

- *Mixed incontinence:* a combination of stress and urge incontinence

- *Functional incontinence:* the inability to hold urine due to reasons other than lower urinary tract dysfunction or neurological reasons. Functional incontinence could be caused by conditions such as urinary tract infection, psychiatric disorders, or impaired mobility.

Medications known to be associated with resulting urinary incontinence include the following:[23]

- cholinergic or anticholinergic drugs
- alpha-blockers
- over-the-counter allergy medications
- betamimetics
- sedatives
- muscle relaxants

- diuretics

- angiotensin-converting enzyme (ACE) inhibitors

Conventional medical treatment of urinary incontinence is similar to that of OAB. In addition, some surgeries can be used to reduce urinary flow through the urethral outlet.

HOLISTIC HELP FOR MALE URINARY PROBLEMS

In addition to treating BPH as described in Chapter 2, the following herbal extracts have been shown to be clinically and scientifically effective for men with OAB and urinary incontinence.

Urox

Urox is an herbal blend that has been a game changer in my practice. When I started using it several years ago, I was stunned by how well it helped men and women with overactive bladder problems as well as mild to moderate cases of urinary incontinence. For the male patients I treat with BPH, I almost always prescribe Urox in addition to herbal prostate formulas, since urinary symptoms improve much more quickly and effectively overall.

The formula consists of concentrated extracts of *Crataeva nurvala* stem bark, *Equisetum arvense* stem, and *Lindera aggregata* root.

- *Crataeva nurvala* is the herb of choice in Ayurvedic medicine for urinary disorders.[24] Research demonstrates that *Crataeva nurvala* significantly decreases residual urine volume and normalizes the tone of the bladder.[25]

- *Equisetum arvense* (horsetail) has a traditional use of treating urinary incontinence and bedwetting in children. Animal research has shown that *Equisetum* influences bladder activity with a relaxant effect.[26] Other researchers credit the benefits for OAB to *Equisetum*'s silica content.[27]

- *Lindera aggregata* has a traditional use in Chinese medicine for frequent urination and incontinence.[28]

A 2018 randomized, double-blind, placebo-controlled trial involved 150 men and women with OAB and urinary incontinence who were given Urox or placebo. After 8 weeks, those taking Urox had significantly fewer episodes of nocturia and lower symptoms of urgency and total incontinence as compared to placebo. The following are some key outcomes of those taking Urox in this remarkable study:[29]

- 61 percent reduction in urinary urgency

- normalization of bladder symptoms for excessive day frequency reported by 60 percent of the Urox group as compared to 11 percent of the control

- 47 percent reduction in nocturia, and total average day frequency returned to normal (less than eight times in 24 hours)

- total remission of nocturia symptoms reported by 24 percent of the Urox group as compared to 2 percent of the control

- 56 percent reduction in urge urinary incontinence

- 67 percent reduction in stress urinary incontinence

- reduced pad usage to one or fewer per day (precautionary purposes only) reported by 75 percent of the Urox group

- willingness to continue treatment expressed by 77 percent of the Urox group as compared to 29 percent of the control

Recommendation: 840 mg Urox daily

Safety: No significant side effects were observed in those taking Urox.

Pumpkin Seed Oil

Pumpkin seed oil from *Cucurbita maxima* was shown in a 12-week study to significantly reduce the degree of OAB in men and women.[30] The dose used in this study was 10 grams of extracted pumpkin seed oil daily. In another study, pumpkin seed oil from *Cucurbita pepo* was shown to significantly improve urinary dysfunction in more than 2,000 men suffering from BPH.[31]

Another randomized, double-blind, placebo-controlled study demonstrated the effectiveness of a pumpkin seed extract (from *Cucurbita pepo*) and soy germ combination in 120 women suffering from OAB. After 12 weeks, those taking this product had a significant reduction in urinary frequency, urgency, incontinence frequency, maximum urgency score, nighttime urination frequency, and OAB symptom score.[32]

Recommendation: Dose depends on type of extract being used. Take as directed on label.

Safety: The treatment was found to be safe with no adverse events.

Cranberry

Many people think of cranberry as a preventive treatment for urinary tract infections. However, a six-month, randomized, double-blind, placebo-controlled study involving 134 men over the age of 45 looked at the effect of cranberry fruit powder on LUTS.[33] At six months, the decrease in the International Prostate Symptom Score (IPSS) was significant for those men taking either 250 or 500 mg of cranberry powder (Flowens) compared to placebo. The decrease in score was considered meaningful according to parameters set by the American Urological Association. For men taking the 500 mg capsule, voiding symptoms were significantly reduced compared to placebo. Also, bladder volume was increased considerably, which may be related to improved bladder detrusor activity. A previous study had found that 1500 mg of dried, powdered cranberries taken daily for six months significantly improved the IPSS quality-of-life score and urination parameters while lowering PSA.[34]

Recommendation: 500 mg daily

Safety: The treatment was found to be safe with no changes in blood markers.

DIETARY CHANGES TO AID LUTS

Men with LUTS can be affected by the different foods they eat and the beverages they consume. I advise following the dietary recommendations outlined in Chapter 2 for BPH as well as the guidelines in Chapter 8. You may also want to keep a food diary to see if you notice any correlation between your urinary symptoms and what you eat and drink. Take into consideration some of the guidelines from the Urology Care Foundation and Mayo Clinic:[35]

- cut out carbonated beverages

- cut back on caffeine

- limit alcohol

- avoid artificial sweeteners, some citrus fruits, tomato-based products, chocolate (other than white chocolate), tea, and spicy foods

NATURAL STRUCTURAL APPROACHES TO LUTS

- *Chiropractic or osteopathic care:* Consider having a spinal assessment by a chiropractor or osteopathic doctor. Nerve flow to the bladder comes through nerves that exit from the lower back (T12–S2) and pelvic region (S2–S4). Cervical (neck) misalignments may affect bladder activity due to effects on the autonomic nervous system. Misalignments or subluxations in these regions can imbalance bladder function due to abnormal nerve messaging. Chiropractic or osteopathy may help bladder symptoms through treatments that improve nerve flow from spinal and surrounding tissues that are causing impingement. A study of men and women with low back pain and leg pain in combination with urinary problems had participants undergo chiropractic treatment for one to eight weeks. Participants in the study had significant improvement in overall urinary frequency and incontinence.[36]

- *Physical therapy:* Some physical therapists are specially trained in pelvic floor disorders and can provide therapy for men with LUTS. This can include muscle strengthening exercises, biofeedback, Kegel exercises, and electrical stimulation.

- *Acupuncture:* There is some research that shows acupuncture can improve symptoms of overactive bladder in adults, either by itself or when combined with drugs.[37]

Even if you've been diagnosed with a prostate condition, remember that holistic approaches provide a more powerful platform to address your symptoms and overall health than treating the prostate only.

CHAPTER 4

PROSTATITIS AND CHRONIC PELVIC PAIN SYNDROME

Manny, a pleasant 67-year-old man, came to my clinic after having dealt with chronic prostatitis for the past six months. His urologist had prescribed different antibiotics without benefit; he was still having penile pain and intermittent blood in his urine. For the past week, he had been on a new antibiotic known as doxycycline, and there had been no change.

I recommended Manny undergo a review by the osteopathic doctor in my clinic for pelvic structural imbalances, since this is common with chronic prostatitis. Also, given his symptoms and history of BPH, I recommended a nutraceutical formula for prostate enlargement and inflammation that contained rye pollen extract (a well-studied natural substance to treat chronic prostatitis) and herbs for BPH such as saw palmetto and nettle root. When I followed up with Manny six weeks later, he reported he no longer had blood in his urine or penile pain. I followed up with him two more times over the next six months, and his symptoms did not return. He continues to use the nutraceutical formula for prostate health.

◆ ◆ ◆

Prostatitis is the most common urinary tract problem for men under the age of 50 and the third most common urinary tract problem for men older than 50.[1] It has been estimated that up to 16 percent of men will be diagnosed with prostatitis at some point in their lifetimes![2]

While both prostatitis and BPH can result in an enlarged prostate, prostatitis specifically means inflammation of the prostate gland tissue. The National Institutes of Health (NIH) lists four different syndromes of prostatitis. Proper classification helps guide the right treatment. The four syndromes are as follows:

- I: acute bacterial prostatitis (ABP)

- II: chronic bacterial prostatitis (CBP)

- III: chronic prostatitis and chronic pelvic pain syndrome (CPPS)

- IV: asymptomatic inflammatory prostatitis

The first two categories are straightforward. They result from a bacterial infection that can be treated with antibiotics and/or natural agents that are antibacterial, along with diet and lifestyle changes that make the prostate less hospitable to infection.

Categories III and IV, which make up most of the cases of prostatitis, are more challenging to doctors, since there can be many different causes that require nonantibiotic treatment.[3]

In the following sections I will discuss the symptoms and root causes, as well as the conventional and holistic approaches, for each of the four syndromes. Recommendations for supplements and other integrative treatments should be tailored by an integrative practitioner according to the specifics of each patient. Therefore,

I do not offer specific doses for supplements as I did in Chapters 2 and 3.

I. ACUTE BACTERIAL PROSTATITIS

Approximately 10 percent of all cases of prostatitis are acute and caused by a bacterial infection. Most cases occur in men ages 20 to 40 or those older than 70 years.[4]

The most common symptoms of ABP are pain, prostate enlargement, failure to void, and fever.[5] Pain can occur in the pelvis and pelvic joints and muscles, or in the rectal, prostate, low back, or low abdominal regions. Other symptoms can include chills, fatigue, and vomiting.[6]

Urinary symptoms may include increased frequency, urgency, painful or difficult urination (dysuria), increased nighttime urination frequency (nocturia), hesitancy, weak stream, incomplete voiding, and urethral discharge.

Your doctor can make a diagnosis of ABP based on your signs and symptoms, physical exam (digital rectal exam), urinalysis, and urine culture.

Causes of Acute Bacterial Prostatitis

There are different theories as to how a man's prostate becomes infected with one or more strains of bacteria. The leading theory is known as intraprostatic urinary reflux. This is when urine backs up into the ejaculatory and prostatic ducts. In younger men, the cause is more likely to be from urinary tract infections that spread up the urethra to the prostate following sexual intercourse.[7] Other causes include infections from medical procedures such as prostate biopsy, catheterization, and cystoscopy.[8]

ABP needs to be taken seriously and treated immediately. Besides the worsening of uncomfortable symptoms,
this condition can progress to chronic prostatitis, pyelo-
nephritis (kidney infection), epididymitis (infection of
the epididymis), or chronic pelvic pain syndrome. Also,
there is the risk of an abscess of the prostate and septice-
mia (blood infection).[9] In more severe cases, hospitalization may be required.

Treatment of Acute Bacterial Prostatitis

Conventional treatment: The primary treatment for ABP
is antibiotic therapy and pain medication. Alpha-blockers
may be used to help with urinary flow.

Integrative treatment: To complement antibiotic treatment for faster healing, I add integrative therapies such as
colloidal silver, oregano oil, echinacea, uva ursi, Oregon
grape, goldenseal, homeopathic medicines, intravenous
vitamin C, and medical ozone therapy (intravenous or rectal). For guidance on which adjunctive therapies are right for
you, be sure to discuss your ABP with an integrative doctor.

Dietary recommendations: To prevent fungal overgrowth
and digestive problems associated with antibiotics, I recommend consuming foods containing probiotics (e.g.,
yogurt, kefir, kombucha, sauerkraut, miso, tempeh, kimchi) as well as probiotic supplements. I have patients take
the probiotics two hours before or after antibiotics are
taken. It's also best to follow a diet low in simple sugars
to reduce inflammation and avoid immune suppression at
this time. The modified Mediterranean diet, as given in
Chapter 8 and the Appendix, is a good choice.

OZONE THERAPY

Numerous studies have demonstrated that the use of low-dose ozone as a medical treatment can be effective in the treatment of infectious agents. Ozone has been shown to inactivate pathogens such as bacteria, fungi, and viruses as well as activate the immune system.[10] The use of ozone to treat infections is common among medical professionals in Germany, Russia, and Cuba, as well as integrative doctors in the United States.

II. CHRONIC BACTERIAL PROSTATITIS

When an infection lasts three months or longer and repeated cultures grow the same bacterial strain, it becomes known as CBP.[11] It typically occurs in men 36 to 50 years of age. The risk factors are the same as those for ABP; about 5 percent of men with ABP progress to CBP.[12]

Your doctor can make a diagnosis of CBP based on your signs and symptoms, physical exam (digital rectal exam), and urine and prostatic fluid culture. While diagnosis is often confirmed with bacterial cultures of urine or prostatic fluid, testing may have false negatives, so a patient may still respond to antibiotic therapy.[13]

Treatment of Chronic Bacterial Prostatitis

Conventional treatment: The conventional treatment for CBP is the same as for ABP and usually involves an antibiotic from the fluoroquinolone family.[14] Additional pharmaceutical therapy may include pain medication and alpha-blockers to help symptoms.[15]

Integrative treatment: Antibiotic resistance and the bacterial production of biofilm can make CBP challenging to treat.[16] Biofilm is a type of slimy membrane that microbes like bacteria secrete to protect them from the body's immune system and to resist antibiotics. Agents that have the ability to break down biofilm include black cumin, silver nanoparticles, ethylenediaminetetraacetate (EDTA), and bismuth.[17] With the addition of one or more of these antibiofilm agents, herbal/nutraceutical therapy for CBP is similar to treatment for ABP. Intravenous vitamin C and medical ozone therapy (intravenous or rectal) can also be used as an adjunct to antibiotic treatment. Of course, you should be under the care of an integrative doctor when using adjunctive therapies for CBP.

In support of the combination of natural approaches with antibiotic therapy, the medical journal *BJU International* states that "phytotherapy [plant therapy] has a modest beneficial effect on symptom improvement in CBP . . . and may be considered as a treatment option in treatment-refractory patients."[18] Furthermore, a study published in the *International Journal of Antimicrobial Agents* studied the effects of natural compounds (saw palmetto, nettles, and the combination of quercetin and curcumin) on 143 men with CBP.[19] All the men received the antibiotic prulifloxacin for 14 days, with one group receiving the natural compounds as well while the other group received only the antibiotic. After one month, 89.6 percent of the group receiving both treatments reported no symptoms related to CBP, as compared to 27 percent of the antibiotics-only group.

Dietary recommendations: To prevent fungal over-growth and digestive problems associated with antibiotics, I recommend consuming foods containing probiotics (e.g., yogurt, kefir, kombucha, sauerkraut, miso, tempeh, kimchi) as well as probiotic supplements. I have patients take the probiotics two hours before or after antibiotics are taken.

III. CHRONIC PROSTATITIS AND CHRONIC PELVIC PAIN SYNDROME

This category involves chronic pelvic pain in men where there is no bacterial prostatitis. The terms *chronic prostatitis, chronic nonbacterial prostatitis,* and *chronic pelvic pain syndrome* all refer to the same condition and are used interchangeably. (I'll be using the acronym CPPS to refer to this condition, although it's important to note that some studies use the acronym CP or CP/CPPS.) The pain is associated with urination and/or pain in the groin, genitalia, or perineum (the area between the anus and scrotum).[20] While no bacteria are found with urinalysis, there can be excess white blood cells or bacteria with testing and culture of prostatic secretions.[21]

This diagnosis needs to meet these three criteria:[22]

1. long-standing symptoms, with a significant number related to structures located within the area of the prostate gland

2. no objective explanation for the patient's symptoms can be identified by doctors

3. no satisfactory treatment for the patient's symptoms

Anxiety, stress, and depression may be part of the symptom picture.[23] In addition, research shows that the prevalence of erectile dysfunction in men with CPPS is between 31.5 and 48.3 percent, which is much higher than in the general population. Studies have shown that the worse the pain symptoms and stress perception are, the worse the erectile dysfunction is.[24]

The Underlying Causes of CPPS

CPPS is a diagnosis of exclusion. This means that other possible diseases are ruled out before making the diagnosis of CPPS. As with the previous cases of prostatitis, there is often a physical examination involving a digital rectal exam, as well as a PSA blood test, urine culture, and possibly imaging studies of the kidneys, ureter, or bladder.

Pelvic floor dysfunction, problems with the proper tightening and relaxing of the pelvic floor muscles, can play a significant role in CPPS. The pelvic floor primarily functions as a sling of muscles found from the coccyx region at the back to the pubic bone at the front. These muscles support the pelvic organs, such as the bladder and bowel, and protect them from external damage. These muscles can become weak or imbalanced from injuries, excessive weight, surgeries, and other reasons.[25]

From a conventional viewpoint, the cause of CPPS is often not clear. According to the Urology Care Foundation, it may be associated with stress, nerve inflammation or irritation, injuries, prior urinary tract infections, pelvic floor muscle tension, prostate stones, urethral stricture (narrowing of the urethra) or scar tissue, prostate cancer, or BPH. Research from 28 Italian urological centers studied men between the ages of 25 and 50 years with CPPS. They found that the prevalence of this condition was closely associated with cigarette smoking, a high-caloric diet with low fruit and vegetable consumption, constipation, intestinal gas, slow digestion, a sexual relationship with more than one partner, and coitus interruptus (sexual intercourse in which the penis is withdrawn before ejaculation).[26]

Research shows that doctors are often confused and frustrated in treating CPPS.[27] This is because many doctors, including urologists, focus only on bacterial causes. More than 90 percent of cases of CPPS, however, are not associated with significant bacterial infection.[28] One of the emerging underlying factors for CPPS is in fact fungal infection. In a urological study involving 1,000 male patients (average age 34) who did not respond to antibiotic and alpha-blocker therapy for prostatitis and were experiencing CPPS, an incredible 80 percent of cases saw improvement from an antifungal regimen! The men were prescribed a low-carbohydrate diet, urine alkalinization, and the antifungal drug fluconazole.[29]

Treatments for Chronic Prostatitis and Chronic Pelvic Pain Syndrome

Conventional treatment: The conventional approach to CPPS usually involves medications. Oftentimes antibiotics will be tried in case there is a bacterial infection that could not be diagnosed. If this treatment fails, then muscle relaxants, alpha-adrenergic blocking agents, nonsteroidal anti-inflammatory agents, alpha-blockers, benzodiazepines, muscle relaxants, gabapentin, tricyclic antidepressants, and other symptom-relieving medications may be used.[30]

Integrative treatment: Integrative therapies go beyond the simplified Western medical model and address multiple causes of CPPS. In doing so, they often offer greater relief of symptoms than conventional therapies alone. Support for this approach is reflected in a recent article in the *Canadian Urological Association Journal*: "There is little downside to considering phytotherapy (particularly quercetin and cernilton) as part of one's multimodal treatment plan. There are few significant side effects (apart from cost) to consider and they have been shown to be more efficacious than placebo in randomized controlled studies."[31] Regardless, the American Urological Association states "There is no evidence that herbs and supplements improve prostatitis."[32] So it is important to find an integrative doctor who is willing to look at all the latest research on herbal extracts.

I have seen many men whose CPPS did not improve with their urologist's antibiotic treatment plan respond well to pharmaceutical and natural antifungal therapies such as oregano oil, caprylic acid, berberine, pau d'arco, biotin, olive leaf, clove, and probiotics. Antifungal/anti-candida formulas are commonly available in health food stores and from integrative practitioners.

Keep in mind that after multiple rounds of antibiotics, one is predisposed to developing fungal infections (gut and prostate). Friendly flora throughout the urinary and prostatic systems are part of the immune system's protection against the overgrowth of fungi. Antibiotics indiscriminately destroy friendly flora and make organs and tissues susceptible to fungal infiltration. As the Johns Hopkins website notes, "Taking antibiotics can also cause an overgrowth of yeast. That's because antibiotics kill the healthy bacteria in your body that normally keep the yeast in balance. . . . Anyone can get a yeast infection."[33]

Many of the following supplements I recommend would be categorized as flavonoids, which have nerve-protective and anti-inflammatory effects. A 2019 study published in the *Journal of the National Medical Association* reviewed studies using plant flavonoids, including quercetin, Cernilton, saw palmetto, curcumin extract, calendula extract, and combination products, to treat CPPS. This meta-analysis showed that flavonoids could significantly improve patients' quality of life. Also, patients given antibiotics along with flavonoids benefitted from a lower recurrence rate and improved quality of life compared to those receiving antibiotics alone.[34]

- *Rye pollen:* One of the best supplements to take for the treatment and prevention of prostatitis is rye pollen extract. Commercial products used in studies usually included the brands Graminex, Cernilton, and Cernitin. This extract is a phenomenal natural agent that resolves chronic CPPS in a significant number of men.

  Rye pollen contains a number of naturally occurring components such as amino acids, carbohydrates, lipids, vitamins, phytosterols, and minerals. The known mechanisms of action include a relaxation effect on the smooth muscles of the bladder and urethra, strong anti-inflammatory effects, and antiproliferative effects.[35]

  Several studies have demonstrated that rye pollen extract (Cernilton) improves the symptoms of CPPS, including prostate pain and overall quality-of-life scores.[36] The authors of a review of studies that included randomized controlled trials concluded that rye pollen extracts "appear to be clinically beneficial as indicated by the significant improvements in terms of the NIH-CPSI [National Institutes of Health Chronic Prostatitis Symptom Index) and QoL [quality of life] scores of patients diagnosed with CPPS. Moreover, this therapeutic approach has an excellent safety profile with limited reported adverse effects."[37]

One study published in the *British Journal of Urology* looked at the effects of a commercial rye pollen extract on 90 men with CPPS. Cernilton was well tolerated by 97 percent of patients. Patients' symptoms, as well as laboratory tests and doctor evaluations after three and six months, indicated favorable results in men who did not have complicating factors: 78 percent of the men had a favorable response, 36 percent were reported cured of their symptoms, and 42 percent improved significantly, with improvements to urinary flow rate and other objective measurements.[38]

- *Saw palmetto:* Saw palmetto also shows promise in treating CPPS when used in combination with other supplements. One study compared the effectiveness and safety of saw palmetto plus the nutrients selenium and lycopene to that of saw palmetto alone for the treatment of CPPS. (The CPPS in this study was IIIa, meaning that inflammation of the prostate was involved, which is indicated by the presence of excess white blood cells in the prostatic secretions.) The study involved 102 men who were randomized to take one of the two treatments for eight weeks. While there was significant improvement in both groups, there was more improvement in the combination product group, as measured by the NIH-CPSI.[39]

The effectiveness of saw palmetto was compared to that of rye pollen in one recent study that had subjects with CPPS take either 320 mg saw palmetto extract or a combination product of flower pollen extract and B vitamins. At the end of the six-week study, researchers concluded that the flower pollen extract/B vitamin formulation was more effective, although both groups reported an improvement in the quality-of-life scores and symptoms. In the combination group, the International Prostate Symptom Score (IPSS) mean score was statistically reduced by up to 82 percent. The authors noted that saw palmetto typically takes more than six weeks to achieve a therapeutic effect, and so this could be a reason that benefits of saw palmetto alone were not as significant as those of the combination product.[40]

• *Quercetin:* Quercetin is another nutraceutical used by integrative doctors for the treatment of CPPS. This flavonoid is found naturally in foods such as onions, kale, broccoli, apples, berries, scallions, and teas.[41] It is also an antioxidant that reduces inflammatory free radicals and inhibits the production of inflammatory chemicals.[42]

In one study, men with CPPS were randomized in a double-blind fashion to receive 500 mg quercetin twice daily or placebo for one month. Those taking quercetin had a significant improvement in symptom scores as compared to those taking placebo. In a follow-up study, 15 additional men received quercetin as well as bromelain and papain to enhance quercetin absorption. Eighty-two percent of the men had at least a 25 percent improvement in their symptom score. The authors concluded that quercetin "is well tolerated and provides significant symptomatic improvement in most men with chronic pelvic pain syndrome."[43]

The effectiveness of quercetin was compared to that of rye pollen in a recent study that had subjects take either 500 mg quercetin twice a day or two capsules a day of a combination product of flower pollen extract and B vitamins.[44] Both groups had similar scores according to the International Prostate Symptom Score (IPSS). However, the group taking the combination product had better quality-of-life scores.

- *Traditional Chinese Medicine:* Traditional Chinese Medicine relies heavily on Chinese herbal formulas for the treatment of many diseases, including CPPS. A review of studies analyzed Danggui Beimu Kushen Wan (DBKW), a classic formula that was developed 1,800 years ago for patients with difficult urination.[45] Researchers found that DBKW used alone or in addition to antibiotics significantly reduced symptom scores. Consult with a licensed practitioner in Traditional Chinese Medicine for patient-specific herbal therapies.

Dietary recommendations: The treatment of CPPS must include dietary changes. As mentioned, a diet restricted in simple carbohydrates is critical. A modified Mediterranean diet (restricted grains) or an antifungal diet, such as the Kaufmann diet, are beneficial. They reduce prostate inflammation and starve infections of the prostate, especially fungal infections.

Food sensitivities may trigger pain in some men with CPPS. In one study of men with CPPS, 47.4 percent reported that consumption of certain items aggravated their pelvic pain symptoms. The most aggravating items reported on the questionnaire were spicy foods, coffee, hot peppers, alcohol, tea, and chili. Items that provided relief included psyllium fiber, water, and herbal teas. Make sure to keep a food diary and note if any foods are worsening your own pelvic pain symptoms. Also, make sure to drink 50 ounces or more of purified water daily.[46]

For more information on a healthy prostate diet, see Chapter 8 and the Appendix.

Physical medicine: Physical medicine can be beneficial for the treatment of CPPS. I recommend men with chronic pelvic pain work with a health-care provider such as an osteopathic physician, chiropractor, acupuncturist, or physical therapist. This is because tight muscles and nerve inflammation, which also reduce blood flow, can be root causes of CPPS. Pelvic floor strengthening exercises may be part of the physical treatment for pelvic pain.

- *Acupuncture:* Acupuncture, which is an essential component of Traditional Chinese Medicine, is a therapy that involves inserting needles through the skin to stimulate specific points. It has been shown in several studies to benefit men with CPPS. A 32-week study published in the *Journal of Urology* found that acupuncture was effective for CPPS.[47] Consult with a licensed acupuncturist to explore the safe and effective use of acupuncture.

- *Myofascial trigger point assessment and release therapy and paradoxical relaxation therapy:* Myofascial trigger point therapy is a technique in which one applies pressure or other stimulation to "trigger points" in affected muscles and tissues. Paradoxical relaxation is a cognitive therapy that trains the nervous system to self-regulate and release pelvic muscle tension.

  Research by a team (urologist, physiotherapist, and psychologist) from Stanford treated 138 men with CPPS who did not respond to conventional therapy. The men were treated for at least one month with myofascial trigger point assessment and release therapy and paradoxical relaxation therapy. Moderate or marked improvement was reported in 72 percent of the treated patients.[48]

- *Osteopathy:* Osteopathic treatments are hands-on techniques that move a patient's muscles and joints.[49] This therapy has produced promising results in CPPS sufferers.

In one study, 35 men with CPPS ages 29 to 70 were allocated to osteopathic treatments or a placebo group. Researchers found that osteopathic treatment was significant in its benefits compared to placebo, which did not produce much change in the men's prostate symptom scores.[50]

- *Biofeedback/neurofeedback therapy:* As with many conditions, your pelvic pain may be significantly influenced by how you handle stress, which can cause tight muscles. Working with a counselor or biofeedback/neurofeedback specialist can help to relax the pelvic floor muscles and reduce your pain.

IV. ASYMPTOMATIC INFLAMMATORY PROSTATITIS

This category refers to inflammation of the prostate without a man having any symptoms. It is usually diagnosed when a man is being evaluated for an elevated PSA level or infertility and white blood cells are found in a sperm analysis.[51]

The condition is likely caused by a bacterial or viral infection which then cause an allergic reaction to seminal fluid and urine that drain poorly and reflux into the prostate tissue, causing inflammation.[52] This chronic inflammation can lead to tissue damage and enlargement, which can then progress to symptomatic symptoms common with BPH.[53]

There is no set conventional treatment, but non-steroidal anti-inflammatory drugs and PDE inhibitors may be prescribed.[54]

❖ ❖ ❖

In conclusion, prostatitis and chronic pelvic pain syndrome are problematic for many men. Other than acute bacterial prostatitis, I find that the holistic therapies described in this chapter are generally much more effective than what conventional medicine has to offer.

CHAPTER 5

PROSTATE CANCER

At 67 years of age, Paul looked quite vital when I first saw him in my office. He told me that he had a low-grade prostate cancer and was declining surgery or any conventional treatment. He requested I provide nutritional and holistic support. It has been six years since we started working together, and Paul's localized prostate tumor has not increased substantially.

◆ ◆ ◆

Many of my male patients over the age of 60 are wary of the words "prostate cancer." There is a reason this disease is on their radar: in the U.S., it is the second most common cancer, outranked only by skin cancer. One in nine men will develop prostate cancer during their lifetimes.[1] For many years, new cases of prostate cancer were declining in America, but recent statistics have shown that the incidence has increased.[2]

Although prostate cancer is the second leading cause of cancer death in American men (behind lung cancer), most men do not die from it. In fact, it has a five-year survival rate of 98 percent.[3] Newer studies have demonstrated that active surveillance is a viable option in older men with prostate cancer, in contrast to invasive conventional cancer therapies. Also, several studies demonstrate the preventive ability of diet and lifestyle factors that dramatically reduce prostate cancer risk and death. In this chapter, you will discover the nutritional and holistic protocols that can be used for prevention, as well as integrative programs to use if you have prostate cancer.

CAUSES AND RISK FACTORS

Prostate cancer, like other cancers, involves uncontrolled cell division. If not treated early, this results in metastasis, spreading into surrounding tissues or other areas of the body. Cancer of the prostate is almost always adenocarcinoma, which means that the cancer occurs in glandular tissues. Most prostate cancers grow slowly, but some are aggressive and spread quickly. Proper medical assessment is necessary to identify your own risk.

There are a number of risk factors that have been studied in regard to prostate cancer. The following risk factors may increase a man's risk of prostate cancer:[4]

- *Age:* The incidence of prostate cancer increases with age, especially after age 50. More than 80 percent of prostate cancers are diagnosed in men who are 65 and older.

- *Location:* North American or northern European locations have higher prostate cancer rates.

- *Family history:* Approximately 20 percent of all prostate cancers are familial, meaning they occur in a family. Familial prostate cancer is due to shared genes as well as shared environmental or lifestyle factors. However, hereditary prostate cancer accounts for about 5 percent of cases. Cases of hereditary cancer stem from gene mutations passed down from one generation to the next.

- *Environmental toxins:* Agent Orange, an herbicide notoriously used during the Vietnam War, was found to increase the risk of prostate cancer, among other cancers. There is also evidence that firefighters have a greatly increased risk of cancer, including prostate cancer, as compared to the general population due to their increased exposure to toxic chemicals.

- *Eating habits:* A diet high in animal fat, especially dairy products, may increase prostate cancer risk. However, a diet high in vegetables, fruits, and legumes may lower the risk. Research demonstrates that the Mediterranean diet is protective against prostate cancer.

- *Obesity:* Men who are obese are at higher risk of getting more aggressive prostate cancer.

- *Race:* African American men seem to be at higher risk, although the reasons are not clear.

- *Smoking:* Smoking does not seem to be a risk factor for low-risk prostate cancer but may be a risk factor for aggressive prostate cancer.

THE DIAGNOSIS OF PROSTATE CANCER

Be sure that your doctor knows whether there is a history of prostate cancer within your family so they can advise you as to whether to receive genetic testing. Hereditary cancers are caused by what is known as germline mutation, meaning there is a mutation in a gene that can be passed on. Somatic mutations—mutations that occur only in affected cells and cannot be passed on to children—can also be involved in prostate cancer. Approximately 89 percent of metastatic castration-resistant prostate cancer tumors (prostate cancer that does not respond to androgen deprivation therapy) contain somatic mutations, while about 9 percent occur due to germline mutations.[5] An oncologist can test for both somatic and germline mutations.

Here is a typical testing scenario in the diagnosis of prostate cancer. Many doctors order a prostate-specific antigen (PSA) blood test as part of a screening physical for middle-aged and older men. If PSA levels are mildly elevated, the doctor may request the patient avoid sexual intercourse and bike riding for two or more days and then retest the PSA.

A doctor may perform a DRE as part of a screening physical. This involves inserting a gloved, lubricated finger into the rectum to palpate (feel) the prostate for any unusual bumps or hardness that may suggest cancer. (If the patient feels pain or tenderness, it may indicate prostatitis.) In a DRE, the back part of the prostate gland, where most prostate cancers begin, is palpated. The front portion is not palpable. The DRE is less effective than the PSA test at screening for prostate cancer. If the doctor finds a suspicious hardness or bump, then a PSA test may be ordered. (The blood draw for a PSA test will be scheduled on another day because a DRE may increase PSA levels.)[6]

A DRE and PSA test are generally the first two steps taken in the diagnosis of prostate cancer. If either of these situations brings up something of concern, further testing will be ordered, which can involve special PSA-type tests. The actual diagnosis of prostate cancer, however, is made only with a prostate biopsy, which generally involves imaging of the prostate with transrectal ultrasound or MRI.[7] Both special PSA-type tests and prostate biopsies will be described in the sections that follow.

DISCOVERER OF PSA CLAIMS IT IS AN UNRELIABLE TEST

Dr. Richard J. Ablin, the scientist who first discovered PSA in 1970, did an interesting interview on the conventional medical website Medscape.[8] Dr. Ablin discovered PSA was elevated in men with prostate cancer as well as a variety of benign conditions, such as BPH. He thought elevated PSA levels may be useful in monitoring and predicting a recurrence of prostate cancers that were thought to be in remission. In 1994, however, the FDA approved the PSA test not only for prostate cancer recurrence but also as a possible predictor of prostate cancer. Dr. Ablin was dismayed by the FDA approval for the PSA test for mass screenings, calling it a "public health disaster" and noting it has a *78 percent false positive rate*. Dr. Ablin feels the approval of the use of the PSA test for screening asymptomatic men was due to "fear and money."

I should note this interview was in 2014 and there have been additional studies on PSA since then, which have been inconclusive. For example, a 2019 article published by the *Journal of the National Comprehensive Cancer Network* states that in recent years, prostate cancer incidence and deaths, as well as the incidence of met-astatic disease, have increased. The authors believe this may be due to declines in the rates of early detection, biopsies, diagnoses of localized prostate cancer, and radical prostatectomy since the U.S. Preventive Services Task Force recommended against generalized PSA screenings in 2012.[9]

THE CONTROVERSIAL PSA TEST

The PSA test has been controversial for several years now. PSA is a protein made in the prostate and released along with prostatic fluid to liquefy semen after ejaculation; it provides sperm cells protection and aids motility and fertility. For the past 30 years, this test has been used as an initial screening test for prostate diseases, including prostate cancer.

There is evidence that screening men with PSA testing can reduce prostate cancer deaths, but the testing also increases the risk of harm from overdetection and overtreatment. For example, a man may have elevated PSA due to a very small, slow-growing tumor that may never cause symptoms or metastasize, and so poses little risk to his life. Research shows that increased PSA testing may lead to overtreatment such as unnecessary surgery and radiation therapy that cause side effects such as urinary incontinence, bowel function problems, erectile dysfunction, and infection.[10] A large, randomized clinical trial of more than 400,000 men aged 50 to 60 years compared one group who underwent just one PSA test screening to men who had none. The researchers followed up after 10 years and found that the single PSA screening detected more prostate cancer cases and yet had no significant effect on prostate cancer mortality. The authors of the study noted that the diagnostics of prostate cancer are changing with advances in imaging as well as genetic testing and other types of blood tests, noting, "A PSA test alone with transrectal ultrasound–guided biopsy may no longer be the standard of care in the early detection of prostate cancer."[11]

Different countries offer different recommendations for PSA screening. For example, the United Kingdom does not advocate PSA screening. However, the U.S. Preventive Services Task Force recommends that men between the ages of 55 and 69 reach an individualized decision after a discussion about the pros and cons with their physicians.[12]

The American Cancer Society (ACS) notes that the chance of having prostate cancer increases as PSA level rises. However, there is no specific cutoff point that can tell if a man has prostate cancer or not. Most labs have a cutoff point of 4 ng/mL, although some have 2.5 or 3 as their guideline. If your results are above that level, your doctor will order further testing to confirm prostate cancer. The ACS notes some other interesting statistics for different PSA levels:[13]

- *Less than 4:* 15 percent of these men would be found to have prostate cancer if a biopsy were done

- *Between 4 and 10:* 25 percent chance of prostate cancer

- *More than 10:* more than 50 percent chance of prostate cancer

It is important to be aware of a number of factors that raise the PSA level that are not related to prostate cancer. These include a diagnosis of BPH or prostatitis, older age, and certain medications such as testosterone. Ejaculation or riding a bicycle may also raise PSA levels for a short time, which is why abstaining from ejaculation for one or two days before testing produces the most accurate results. Urological procedures such as cystoscopy or prostate biopsy, and possibly DREs, may also raise PSA levels, which is why doctors generally schedule the blood draw for a different day.[14]

You should also be aware of treatments that may lower PSA levels. It is possible a man may have prostate cancer but a treatment he is taking is lowering his PSA so that an elevation is not as detectable. Examples include BPH medications such as finasteride (Proscar or Propecia) or dutasteride (Avodart), certain supplements and herbal remedies, aspirin, statins (cholesterol-lowering drugs), and thiazide diuretics.[15] Always tell your doctor what medications and supplements you are taking so this can be accounted for if a PSA test is done.

Variations of PSA Testing

If a man has an abnormal PSA test due to elevation (usually >4 ng/mL), then additional PSA-type tests may be ordered before more invasive and costly testing, such as imaging studies or biopsy, is done. The following are specialized PSA tests as described by the American Cancer Society[16] and National Cancer Institute:[17]

- *Percent-free PSA:* There are two major forms of PSA in the blood: one that is attached to protein carriers (also known as bound PSA) and another that circulates unattached (free PSA). The percent-free PSA is the ratio of the amount of free PSA compared to the total PSA level. The percentage of free PSA is lower in men who have prostate cancer than in men who do not.

Doctors may order this test if the PSA test is in the borderline range of between 4 and 10 ng/mL. If the percent-free PSA is low (usually 10 percent or less, although some will advise testing at 10 to 25 percent), then a doctor is more likely to order imaging or biopsy testing.

- *Complexed PSA:* This test measures the amount of bound PSA. It is not a common test, especially as compared to checking the percent-free PSA.

- *Prostate Health Index (PHI):* This test combines the values of total PSA, free PSA, and proPSA (a precursor protein of PSA that is more strongly associated with prostate cancer than with BPH).

- *4Kscore:* This test combines the results of total PSA, free PSA, intact PSA (one of three forms of free PSA), human kallikrein-2 (an enzyme produced by prostate cells), and other factors.

- *PSA velocity:* This is a measure of how quickly the PSA level rises over time. (ACS guidelines do not recommend using PSA velocity as part of screening for prostate cancer.)

- *PSA density:* Since men with larger prostate glands have higher PSA levels, the PSA density takes into account the size (volume) of the prostate based on transrectal ultrasound and divides the PSA number by the prostate volume. A higher PSA density suggests a greater likelihood of cancer.

PROSTATE BIOPSY

The definitive test for prostate cancer is a prostate biopsy, in which small samples of the prostate are removed by your urologist and analyzed by a pathologist. An imaging test such as transrectal ultrasound, MRI, or a combination of the two is used to view the prostate while a needle is inserted through the wall of the rectum or the perineum to take samples from multiple areas of the prostate. Prostate biopsies are reported as negative, positive, or suspicious (i.e., abnormal but potentially noncancerous).[18]

Newer genetic tests, including SelectMDx and ExoDx, can aid in the prediction of your likelihood of prostate cancer, which can help you and your care provider decide whether a prostate biopsy is necessary.

The following information should help you understand what you'll find on your pathology report.

Gleason Grades, Gleason Sums, and Score Groupings

A positive biopsy is given a grade based on how the cancer appears under a microscope. The more abnormal the cells look, the higher the grade. The prostate cancer grade is known as the Gleason grade. A Gleason grade of 1 to 5 is assigned based on how much the cancer appears like normal prostate tissue:[19]

- Grade 1 is cancer that looks like normal prostate tissue.

- Grade 5 denotes cells and their growth patterns that appear very abnormal.

- Grades 2 through 4 have features between these extremes.

It is important to know that prostate cancers often have tissue areas with different grades, and therefore grades are given to the two areas that comprise most of the cancer. The two grades added together provide the Gleason score, also known as the Gleason sum. Sometimes three grades from more than two areas are used in calculating this score.[20]

Your report will generally show three numbers as part of your Gleason score. The first number is the most common Gleason grade in the tumor. For example, a Gleason score of 3 + 4 = 7 means most of the tumor is grade 3, a smaller part is grade 4, and added together creates a Gleason score of 7. Other ways that this Gleason score might be written out are Gleason 7/10, Gleason 7 (3 + 4), or combined Gleason grade of 7.

There are three main groups for the Gleason score:

- *Gleason score 6 or less:* well differentiated, or low-grade. These cancers tend to grow and spread slowly.

- *Gleason score 7:* moderately differentiated, or intermediate-grade. These cancers are likely to grow and spread quickly.

- *Gleason score 8 to 10:* poorly differentiated, or high-grade. Cancers with a score of 9 or 10 are twice as likely to grow and spread quickly as those with a score of 8.

Another way doctors assess the Gleason score is through Grade Groups. It is thought these Grade Groups will replace the Gleason score over time, as they are easier for patients to understand, but you will likely receive both scores for now. These groups range from 1 (most likely to grow and spread slowly) to 5 (most likely to grow and spread quickly):[21]

- *Grade Group 1:* Gleason 6 (or less)
- *Grade Group 2:* Gleason 3 + 4 = 7
- *Grade Group 3:* Gleason 4 + 3 = 7
- *Grade Group 4:* Gleason 8
- *Grade Group 5:* Gleason 9 and 10

Other Notes on a Pathology Report

Biopsy reports usually list the number of biopsy samples that contain cancer (e.g., "8 out of 12"). Each sample of tissue taken is called a *core*. Your report will refer to each core by an identifying number or letter and give each one its own diagnosis. It should describe the percentage of cancer in each of the core samples as well as which side of the prostate (left or right) the cancer is located on if both sides are involved (bilateral).

Prostate biopsies may find cells that look suspicious but not cancerous. This is known as prostatic intraepithelial neoplasia (PIN). There are two main categories:[22]

- *Low-grade PIN:* This pattern of prostate cells appears almost normal. These types of cells are not thought to be related to prostate cancer risk and won't be noted on your report.

- *High-grade PIN:* This pattern of cells looks more abnormal and could indicate a higher likelihood that a man will develop prostate cancer over time. These cases are considered precancerous and may warrant closer monitoring and testing, including more prostate biopsies.

- *ASAP (atypical small acinar proliferation):* This is considered a precancerous state based on a prostate biopsy.

IMAGING TESTS

Imaging tests can be used to evaluate the size of a prostate tumor and to see if it has spread in the body. They are also used to help guide a biopsy or for localized treatments such as brachytherapy or cryotherapy. The following imaging tests are generally used for prostate evaluation and treatment:[23]

- *Transrectal ultrasound (TRUS):* A probe that emits sound waves is inserted into the rectum to image the prostate and evaluate the size and location of a tumor. Another version of this is color Doppler ultrasound, which also provides a sense of blood flow to the tumor. (This may be helpful since tumors often display increased blood flow, or angiogenesis.)

- *Magnetic resonance imaging (MRI):* This type of imaging involves the use of radio waves and magnets to give a detailed picture. Usually a contrast dye is injected into the body for better imaging. An MRI can be used after abnormal prostate tests to see if a biopsy is necessary. It can also be used to see if a prostate cancer has spread in the body to nearby or other structures.

Multiparametric MRI, a newer technique, involves the use of a standard MRI and at least one other type of MRI to assess whether a man may have prostate cancer.

- *MRI/ultrasound fusion guided prostate biopsy:* This involves an MRI scan days or weeks before the biopsy to find abnormal areas of the prostate. Then TRUS is used to view the prostate during the biopsy. The images of the previous MRI are fused with the TRUS for an enhanced view of the prostate.

- *Computed tomography (CT or CAT) scan:* A machine takes X-rays of the inside of the body from different angles. A contrast dye may be injected or taken as a pill or liquid for best results.

- *Positron emission tomography (PET):* This technology involves a machine that evaluates the metabolism of cells of body tissues by analyzing a small amount of a radioactive drug injected into the body. It is often combined with a CT scan, a process known as a PET-CT scan. With cancer there is a higher metabolic activity that can show up on a PET scan.

- *Bone scan:* This test looks for metastasis of prostate cancer to the bones. It involves the injection of a radioactive material that settles in the affected areas of bones. A special camera detects the radioactivity and produces a picture of one's skeleton. An MRI or CT scan may be used to follow up on an abnormal bone scan.

- *Lymph node biopsy:* Biopsies of lymph nodes near the prostate may be done to see if cancer has spread. Also, lymph nodes may be removed and analyzed during surgery for prostate removal (radical prostatectomy).

UNDERSTANDING CONVENTIONAL TREATMENTS

There are a number of conventional treatments available for prostate cancer. The American Society of Clinical Oncology recommends that a patient with cancer have a team of different doctors with various specialties.[24] This makes good sense and should include a doctor trained in science-based integrative and nutritional therapies, as discussed in the next section.

Since most prostate cancers are found at an early stage and are slow growing, most men do not need to be in a hurry to make treatment decisions. You should understand your treatment options and potential side effects. Take the time to seek out integrative doctors and other credentialed holistic providers to form part of your multidisciplinary team.

The following options are recommended by the American Society of Clinical Oncology and the American Cancer Society.[25]

Active Surveillance

Men with very-low-risk prostate cancer have the option of what is termed "active surveillance." This means that they can delay cancer treatment while under the supervision of medical professionals because their cancer is at a stage where it is unlikely to cause harm or decrease life expectancy. One of the main reasons men choose active surveillance is to avoid the potential side effects of prostate cancer therapy, such as erectile dysfunction and incontinence. The Prostate Cancer Foundation notes,

> Over 30% of men have prostate cancers that are so slow growing and "lazy" that Active Surveillance is a better choice than immediate local treatment with surgery or radiation. Of the top 10 most common cancers, prostate cancer is the only one in which so many patients have a slow-growing tumor that does not warrant aggressive immediate treatment.[26]

The American Society of Clinical Oncology supports active surveillance for most men whose prostate cancer has not spread beyond the prostate and who have a Gleason score of 6 or lower. For men under active surveillance, they recommend the following testing schedule:

- A PSA test every 3 to 6 months
- A DRE at least once every year
- Another prostate biopsy within 6 to 12 months of the first, then a biopsy at least every 2 to 5 years

If there are signs of cancer becoming more aggressive or spreading, then treatment is initiated.

Watchful Waiting

Older men who are expected to live less than five years due to serious or life-threatening diseases may choose "watchful waiting" and no conventional treatment. The difference between watchful waiting and active surveillance is that typical testing, such as the PSA, DRE, and biopsies, is not done. If a man is experiencing pain or urinary tract blockage, then treatments such as hormonal suppression may be implemented.

Local Treatments

Local treatments are an option for early-stage prostate cancer. These treatments are less invasive and destroy small prostate tumors but not the whole gland.

- *High-intensity focused ultrasound (HIFU):* Sound waves from an ultrasound probe are used to destroy cancer cells.

- *Cryosurgery (cryotherapy, cryoablation):* A metal probe is inserted into an incision between the rectum and scrotum to freeze and kill cancer cells.

- *Radiation therapy:* This common approach utilizes high-energy rays to kill cancer cells. There are two main types of radiation therapy.
  External beam radiation involves radiation focused on the prostate gland from an outside machine. There are different types of technologies for external beam radiation, including proton beam therapy, which emits

protons instead of X-rays. Side effects from external beam radiation can include bowel problems, urinary problems, erection problems, fatigue, and lymphedema (lymph fluid collecting in an area and causing swelling).

Internal radiation, also known as brachytherapy, involves small radioactive pellets that are placed directly into the prostate tissue. Potential side effects include bowel, urinary, and erectile problems. There is also a small risk the seeds could move and come out.

Chemotherapy

This common type of treatment involves the use of anticancer drugs given orally or injected into a vein. Chemotherapy is often recommended when cancer has spread outside the prostate gland and hormone therapy is ineffective. In most cases, the chemo drug first given is docetaxel combined with the steroid drug prednisone. If docetaxel is not effective, then the chemo drug cabazitaxel is often prescribed.

Common side effects of chemotherapy include hair loss, mouth sores, loss of appetite, nausea and vomiting, diarrhea, infections, bruising, bleeding, and fatigue.

Hormone Therapy

Hormone therapy for prostate cancer is also known as androgen suppression therapy (AST) or androgen deprivation therapy (ADT). Androgens are a group of hormones made primarily by the testicles and adrenal glands that include testosterone and its metabolite dihydrotestosterone (DHT). Lowering levels of these hormones, especially DHT, may reduce the growth effects on prostate cells.

Hormone therapy is typically used if the cancer has spread too far to be effectively treated by surgery or radiation, or if the cancer comes back after surgery or radiation therapy. ADT is also used along with radiation therapy as the initial treatment or, if the patient is at higher risk of a cancer relapse, after treatment. ADT is used before radiation to shrink the cancer to make treatment more effective.

There are a number of different types of hormone therapy:

- *Surgical castration (orchiectomy):* This involves the physical removal of the testicles, which are the glands that produce most of the body's testosterone and DHT.

- *LHRH agonists:* Luteinizing hormone-releasing hormone agonists, also known as LHRH analogs or GnRH agonists, are medications that reduce the testosterone production of the testicles. These drugs are injected or implanted under the skin. Examples include leuprolide (Lupron, Eligard), goserelin (Zoladex), triptorelin (Trelstar), and histrelin (Vantas).

  This treatment is also known as medical castration since androgens are reduced to a level similar to that seen in surgical castration.

- *LHRH antagonists:* This treatment is also a form of medical castration and is given as an injection. It works similarly to LHRH agonists; however, this medication is more effective in lowering testosterone at a quicker rate and

without the flare-ups seen at the beginning
of treatment with an LHRH agonist. One
medication is known as degarelix (Firmagon).

Potential side effects of orchiectomy, LHRH agonists,
and LHRH antagonists include reduced or absent sexual desire, erectile dysfunction, shrinkage of the testicles
and penis, hot flashes, breast tenderness and breast tissue
growth, osteoporosis, anemia, decreased mental sharp-
ness, loss of muscle mass, weight gain, fatigue, increased
cholesterol levels, and depression.

- *Androgen synthesis inhibitors:* Abiraterone
  (Zytiga) blocks an enzyme that the adrenal
  glands and prostate cancer cells use in
  making androgens. This drug is used with
  men who have metastatic prostate cancer
  or cancer that is resistant to treatment
  with LHRH agonists, LHRH antagonists, or
  orchiectomy. The treatment is a daily pill.
  Side effects can include muscle pain, high
  blood pressure, fluid retention, hot flashes,
  and digestive upset.

  Ketoconazole blocks the production of
  androgens by the adrenal glands. It is also
  used if other types of hormone therapy are
  not working with advanced prostate cancer.
  Side effects may include elevated liver
  enzymes, nausea, vomiting, breast tissue
  enlargement, and a skin rash.

- *Androgen receptor inhibitors:* This group of
  oral drugs works by blocking prostate cell
  receptors known as androgen receptors.
  This prevents androgens from fueling tumor

growth. They are most commonly used in addition to orchiectomy or an LHRH agonist. Examples include flutamide (Eulexin), bicalutamide (Casodex), and nilutamide (Nilandron).

Side effects are similar to those given for LHRH agonists, LHRH antagonists, and orchiectomy. However, androgen receptor inhibitors have fewer sexual side effects.

- *Additional antiandrogens:* There are newer antiandrogens that can be used for prostate cancer that is not responding to other forms of hormone therapy or for metastatic prostate cancer. Examples include enzalutamide (Xtandi), apalutamide (Erleada), and darolutamide (Nubeqa).

  Side effects can include diarrhea, fatigue, rash, hot flashes, dizziness, and (rarely) seizures.

Immunotherapy

Immunotherapy, also known as biological therapy, involves the enhancement of the immune system to fight cancer. It can entail the stimulation of one's immune system or the use of substances that mimic immune system components to improve or restore one's immune system, allowing it to seek out and attack cancer cells.

- *Cancer vaccine:* Used to treated advanced, recurrent prostate cancer, this treatment must be created specifically for each person. Sipuleucel-T (Provenge) involves taking white blood cells from the patient that are then sent to a lab and mixed with prostatic acid phosphatase (PAP), a protein from prostate cancer cells. The white blood cells are then given back to the patient by infusion into a vein. Treatments are repeated over time. This treatment helps the immune system to locate and attack prostate cancer.

Side effects may include fever, chills, fatigue, back and joint pain, nausea, and headache.

- *Immune checkpoint inhibitor:* This treatment involves the drug known as pembrolizumab (Keytruda). It blocks a protein, PD-1, that prevents immune cells known as T cells from attacking normal cells in the body. The blocking of PD-1 has an immune-boosting effect against prostate cancer. It is given as an infusion.

  Side effects may include fatigue, cough, nausea, itching, skin rash, decreased appetite, constipation, joint pain, and diarrhea.

Targeted Therapy

This type of treatment involves medications that identify and target cancer cells with little effect on normal cells. Prostate cancer generally involves treatment with PARP inhibitors such as rucaparib (Rubraca) and olaparib (Lynparza). These medications are used to treat cancers that have not responded to androgen deprivation therapy, chemotherapy, or other treatments.

The main mechanism of action with these medications is to block PARP enzymes. These enzymes normally help repair damaged DNA cells, but this treatment makes it difficult for certain mutated prostate cancer cells to repair their DNA, thus helping destroy them.

Side effects of PARP inhibitors can include digestive upset such as nausea, vomiting, constipation, diarrhea, and loss of appetite. Other side effects can include fatigue, anemia, cough, shortness of breath, blood clots, and rarely blood cancers.[27]

INTEGRATIVE TREATMENT

Men with prostate cancer commonly turn to complementary and alternative medicine (CAM). The term *complementary* refers to incorporating treatments such as nutrition, herbs, vitamins, minerals, dietary supplements, and other holistic, nondrug therapies as an addition to standard treatments. Research has shown that men with prostate cancer use CAM due to their "medical history, beliefs about the safety and side effects of CAM compared to standard treatments, and a need to feel in control of their treatment."[28] A review of published research on nutritional and holistic approaches concluded that men with prostate cancer may benefit from lifestyle and complementary therapies along with their conventional care.[29]

Integrative treatment of prostate cancer has many supportive effects for men with this disease. In addition to the goal of enhancing the benefits of conventional treatment and outcome, effects of integrative treatment may include the following:[30]

- combating the side effects of fatigue from chemotherapy or radiation
- helping tissue heal from surgery
- easing anxiety and depression
- improving digestive upset
- alleviating joint and muscle pain
- supporting the immune system and preventing/treating infections
- reducing hot flashes and other hormonal symptoms from hormonal therapies
- regimens for protecting against damage to internal organs, such as the liver and heart
- healing skin burns and rashes
- maintaining a healthy body weight and fat percentage
- supporting detoxification
- supporting gut health

THE IMPORTANCE OF DIET

An increasing number of oncologists are recognizing the value of a proper diet in the prevention and treatment of prostate and other cancers. The health of cells and their DNA is strongly tied to the environment provided by one's nutrition. If you are being proactive in preventing or treating prostate cancer, then it is very important to fuel your body with the right foods that promote a healthy immune system and a good environment for cellular health.

One of the reasons diet is so important is that it a controllable factor that people can modify to reduce inflammation. As is true of virtually every disease, cancer is highly related to a state of inflammation. As the National Cancer Institute notes, "Over time, chronic inflammation can cause DNA damage and lead to cancer."[31]

How effective can diet and lifestyle changes be for prostate cancer? A study published in the *Journal of Urology* in 2005 looked at the effects of diet and lifestyle changes on men with prostate cancer who declined conventional treatment. This one-year study included 93 volunteers who were diagnosed with prostate cancer and had PSA levels of 4 to 10 ng/mL and Gleason scores of less than 7. The men were randomly assigned either to an experimental group that was asked to make dietary and lifestyle changes or to a usual care control group.[32]

The experimental group was given a diet that focused on fruits, vegetables, whole grains, legumes, and soy products. Overall, the diet was lower in fat and low in simple carbohydrates. The experimental group was also given soy protein powder, fish oil (3 grams daily), vitamin E (400 IU daily), selenium (200 mcg daily), and vitamin C (2000 mg daily) and instructed to partake in moderate aerobic exercise (walking 30 minutes, 6 days a week), stress-management techniques, and a one-hour support group. Those following the diet and lifestyle changes had improved PSA levels by an average of 4 percent, while those in the control group had their levels worsen by 6 percent. Also, none of the men in the experimental group required oncology treatment based on their PSA and MRI testing, compared with six men in the control group who did require conventional treatment.[33]

A more recent study published in the *British Journal of Cancer* reported on a study done by a multidisciplinary team of urological surgeons, radiation oncologists, and medical oncologists at MD Anderson Cancer Center. Men who were newly diagnosed with prostate cancer and had a Gleason score of 6 or 7 were monitored twice yearly, and a food questionnaire was completed. At the end of three years, researchers found an inverse relationship between diet quality and risk of Gleason grade progression. In other words, a higher-quality diet that consists of different fiber-rich plant foods and a healthy balance of unsaturated fats, while lower in saturated fats, added sugars, and refined grains, "may be beneficial for men diagnosed with early-stage prostate cancer."[34]

Essentially, any diet that focuses on foods as close as possible to their natural state is optimal. A balance of fats, low intake of refined carbohydrates, and mild-to-moderate intake of protein tends to be the basis of most beneficial diets. Along with the Mediterranean diet, which I highly recommend, additional diets for men with prostate cancer to consider with the help of a nutritionist or integrative doctor include vegetarianism, the Kaufmann diet, and ketogenic diets (for short-term use).

The Mediterranean Diet

While many different diets are recommended for prostate cancer prevention and treatment, the one that has plenty of solid research behind it is the Mediterranean diet. The Mediterranean diet consists of plenty of plant foods (fruits, vegetables, legumes, nuts, breads, and unrefined cereals); lots of olive oil; moderately high intake of fish; moderate consumption of alcohol; and low consumption of poultry, red meat, and eggs.[35]

Research has shown that countries that follow the traditional Mediterranean diet, especially southern European countries, have lower prostate cancer incidence and mortality compared with other European countries.[36] In one study following 4,538 men diagnosed with nonmetastatic prostate cancer, it was found that the Mediterranean diet was associated with lower overall mortality.[37] Another study followed 118 men with prostate cancer, along with 238 other men from the same geographical region as a control group. Researchers found that those men who adhered to the Mediterranean diet most closely had a 78 percent lower likelihood of having prostate cancer.[38]

Research has shown that the Mediterranean diet may be more protective against aggressive and advanced prostate cancers.[39] This conclusion was published in the *Journal of Urology*; the researchers found that high adherence to the Mediterranean diet was "specifically associated with a lower risk of Gleason score greater than 6 prostate cancer . . . or with higher clinical stage," whereas the Western dietary pattern did not show any association with reduced prostate cancer risk.[40]

There are many factors that may explain why the Mediterranean diet has anticancer properties. The Mediterranean diet has the following attributes:[41]

- is high in polyphenols, which have antioxidant, anti-inflammatory, and gene-regulating effects
- contains lycopene (as found in tomatoes), a phytochemical that has antioxidant and anti-inflammatory effects

- supports better weight management (obesity and insulin resistance increase cancer risk)
- regulates blood pressure and insulin sensitivity, so one is more resistant to the damaging effects of oxidation, inflammation, and blood vessel abnormalities

For meal planning that includes the Mediterranean diet, see Chapter 8 and the Appendix of this book. And for a more thorough discussion of the integrative treatment of cancer, see my book *Outside the Box Cancer Therapies*.

Green Tea

Green tea is made from the fresh leaves of *Camellia sinensis*. Green tea contains a group of compounds known as polyphenols that are composed of catechins. The major polyphenol in green tea is known as epigallocatechin-3-gallate (EGCG).

Several studies have shown that EGCG exihibits anti-cancer activity. A review of studies published in the journal *Medicine* reviewed a total of seven controlled trials on the preventive effects of green tea on prostate cancer.[42] The researchers of this study found a trend of reduced incidence of prostate cancer for every one cup of green tea consumed per day, and especially with more than seven cups per day consumed.

Recommendation: Drink as many cups of organic green tea as is tolerable or as recommended by your integrative doctor.

Safety: Green tea contains less caffeine than coffee, but patients sensitive to caffeine may require lower amounts. Your oncologist may not want you on higher doses of green tea while undergoing chemotherapy.

MALNUTRITION AND CANCER

For men with prostate cancer, it is important to recognize that a lack of nutrition, or malnutrition, is a problem that affects the majority of people with cancer. If your oncologist dismisses the value of a healthy diet, then it goes against what the science shows.

An article published in the mainstream journal *Oncotarget* stated, "In cancer patients, malnutrition is associated with treatment toxicity, complications, reduced physical functioning, and decreased survival."[43] The same authors found that in an observation study of 1,952 patients with cancer, 51 percent had nutritional impairment, 9 percent were overly malnourished, 43 percent were at risk for malnutrition, and 40 percent were experiencing anorexia (loss of appetite). The study authors also reported that "high prevalence of cancer-related malnutrition and its negative consequences are taken too lightly in most oncology units."

SUPPLEMENTATION

There are a number of supplements that can be used as a complementary therapy for men with prostate cancer. Keep in mind that there is no nutritional supplement that has been shown to cure prostate cancer. However, there are supplements that have shown to boost immunity and reduce the side effects of conventional therapy such as radiation and chemotherapy. The following recommendations for therapeutic use are based on my own experiences with patients with prostate cancer as well as the published literature. Your integrative doctor can help you decide which supplements to use for your particular situation.

Vitamin D

Vitamin D has been shown to have numerous anti-cancer effects, including modulation of proper cell division, apoptosis, activation of tumor-suppression gene p53, inhibition of angiogenesis, inhibition of motility and invasion, and modulation of tumor-associated growth factors.[44] Several population studies have shown a higher risk of prostate cancer or lethal prostate cancer in men living in northern latitudes, where vitamin D intake is low (due to decreased exposure to sunlight, which stimulates vitamin D production).[45] In a meta-analysis involving 7,808 men with prostate cancer, it was found that "higher 25-hydroxyvitamin D level was associated with a reduction of mortality in prostate cancer patients and vitamin D is an important protective factor in the progression and prognosis of prostate cancer."[46]

Recommendation: 2000 to 5000 IU daily, with a meal. However, dosing is best based on serum vitamin D (25-hydroxyvitamin D) levels. A level of 50 ng/mL is a decent serum vitamin D level.

Safety: Vitamin D is considered to be a safe supplement at regular dosages. Levels can be monitored with blood testing.

Coriolus versicolor

Coriolus versicolor, also known by the common name turkey tail, is the world's most well-studied medicinal mushroom. Several hundred studies have investigated its immune-stimulating and anticancer properties, particularly in "hot-water extracts" where active constituents are extracted by pressing a substance through hot water.

Coriolus contains substances known as beta-glucans that stimulate the immune system, including white blood cells, natural killer cells, and other anticancer chemicals produced by the body.[47] It has also been shown to reduce cell proliferation[48] and increase natural killer cell activity.[49] Moreover, Coriolus has been shown to reduce side effects in people undergoing chemotherapy and radiation treatments.[50]

Recommendation: 2000 to 3000 mg daily of a hot-water extract

Safety: Turkey tail is well tolerated.

Maitake

Maitake (*Grifola frondosa*) is an edible mushroom that is used medicinally as a hot-water extract. It is used in integrative cancer therapy in Asia and North America. Maitake contains unique, immune-boosting beta-glucans.[51]

Maitake has been shown to reduce adverse reactions and pain for those with terminal stage cancer who were undergoing chemotherapy.[52]

Recommendation: The most well-studied maitake products are hot-water extracts, including maitake D-fraction and MD-fraction. Take 0.5 to 1 mg per 2.2 pounds of body weight per day, or 35 to 70 mg of maitake extract daily. It is best taken on an empty stomach.

Safety: Maitake extracts are very safe. A small percentage of users may experience loose stool, which may be alleviated with a lower dose. Those on immunosuppressive drugs should not use maitake without the consent of their physician.

Modified Citrus Pectin

Modified citrus pectin (MCP) is an extract from the peel and pith of citrus fruits. The benefit of MCP is that it binds and inactivates a protein known as galectin-3.[53] Galectin-3 is problematic in that it causes the migration of cancer cells to tissue, aids the formation of blood vessels that supply tumors, prevents cancer cell death, and aids in the metastasis of cancer.[54] MCP interferes with the signaling of galectin-3 and improves immune cell activity.[55]

A 12-month trial of 15 grams daily of MCP supplementation was conducted with 10 men with prostate cancer.[56] These men had not responded well to treatments such as prostatectomy, radiation, or cryosurgery. MCP was shown to significantly slow the rise of prostate-specific antigen (PSA) in 7 out of 10 men (elevated PSA being an indicator of cancer growth).

Also, studies done with human and mouse prostate cancer cells have shown that MCP can inhibit cell proliferation and apoptosis.[57]

Recommendation: Patients with active cancer should take 5 grams, three times daily, with lots of water. For preventative purposes, you can take 5 grams once a day.

Safety: MCP is very safe. One may need to increase the dose over time due to the digestive system getting used to the fiber. This is a type of fiber, so do not ingest with oral medications, as it may decrease their efficacy.

Turmeric

Turmeric (*Curcuma longa*) is a bright-yellow spice that is regularly found in Indian food. It is commonly used as a medicinal agent in Ayurvedic and Asian medicine. It contains a group of compounds known as curcuminoids, among which curcumin is the most researched.

Curcumin has antioxidant, anti-inflammatory, and anti-cancer properties.[58] It also regulates gene expression that affects cancer growth.[59]

While human studies are still underway, according to the Mayo Clinic, "Laboratory and animal research suggests that curcumin may prevent cancer, slow the spread of cancer, make chemotherapy more effective and protect healthy cells from damage by radiation therapy."[60]

Recommendation: Add one teaspoon organic turmeric to a shake or meal daily. For more aggressive use, take 1500 to 3000 mg of a standardized extract as a daily supplement.

Safety: Side effects are minimal. Research has shown that people tolerate up to 8000 mg daily of curcumin for three months with minimal side effects.[61] Turmeric has antiplatelet properties, so lower doses may need to be used for those on anticoagulant therapies.[62]

EXERCISE

For optimal immunity, it is critical for men with prostate cancer or a history of prostate cancer to exercise regularly. There are numerous studies that demonstrate how exercise enhances the immune system. Physical activity may reduce the risk of cancer in one of several ways, including lowering the levels of certain sex hormones, preventing high levels of insulin, reducing inflammation, and controlling weight gain.

Exercise immunology, a relatively new field of science, studies the effects of exercise on the immune system.

Moderate- to vigorous-intensity aerobic exercise for less than 60 minutes has been shown to improve immune activity of many components of the immune system, including natural killer (NK) cells. Also, this type of exercise reduces chemicals that cause inflammation.[63]

There is also the even newer field of exercise oncology. Researchers in this field have conducted more than 1,000 randomized clinical trials. The National Cancer Institute notes that there is evidence that exercise after a diagnosis of prostate cancer is associated with longer survival. The NCI's recommendations include 2.5 hours to 5 hours per week of moderate-intensity exercise or 1.25 to 2.5 hours per week of vigorous activity.[64]

Just a half hour of aerobic exercise three times a week improves quality of life in cancer survivors, including levels of depression, fatigue, and physical function.[65] And according to an interview with Dr. Johnson of Johns Hopkins Medicine, "Several studies suggest that men who take part in regular physical activity are less likely to develop prostate cancer or die from the disease."[66] He notes that one of the big reasons for this beneficial effect is weight loss, since obesity is associated with prostate cancer.

A study of men with prostate cancer found that those men who participated in three or more hours per week of vigorous activity experienced a 61 percent reduced rate of mortality compared with men who participated in less than one hour per week of comparable activity.[67]

Recommendation: 30 to 60 minutes daily of moderate exercise is highly recommended. Resistance training should be included if at all possible to help maintain muscle mass, which often decreases in those with cancer.

COMBAT THE EFFECTS OF STRESS

Numerous studies have shown that how a person perceives and handles stress is connected to that person's susceptibility to and survival from cancer. In one review, researchers found at least 165 studies demonstrating that stress-related psychosocial factors are associated with higher cancer incidence in initially healthy populations. The authors also found hundreds of studies that linked poorer survival rates and higher cancer mortality to these stress-related factors.[68]

When we do not handle stress well, our immune systems become more hospitable to cancer. There are numerous ways to reduce the effects of stress that go beyond exercise, such as proper sleep patterns, humor and laughter, prayer, counseling, biofeedback, and many others. Consistent use of these methods is important for an optimal immune system.

ADDITIONAL INTEGRATIVE THERAPIES

There are a number of other holistic, complementary therapies that integrative oncologists and doctors use to improve quality of life as well as boost immunity. This includes the use of high-dose intravenous vitamin C, CBD/THC, hyperbaric oxygen therapy, medical-grade ozone, acupuncture, and several other therapies. Your integrative doctor can guide you on what therapies match your situation best. (You can also review my book *Outside the Box Cancer Therapies*.)

High-dose intravenous vitamin C (IVC) is the most well-studied and effective integrative therapy for cancer treatment. It is usually given by integrative oncologists and doctors at doses between 25 grams and 100 grams. At my clinic we typically administer 50 grams as the average dosage.

Intravenous vitamin C has been shown to boost anti-cancer activity. A study in the *Proceedings of the National Academy of Sciences of the United States of America* showed that IVC selectively kills cancer cells by delivering hydrogen peroxide to tissues.[69] Other research shows that high-dose intravenous vitamin C significantly reduces inflammation, activates a gene that suppresses tumor formation, and has antiangiogenic effects.[70]

Intravenous vitamin C also improves quality-of-life scores for people undergoing chemotherapy. One review summarizes, "Several recent studies have indicated that intravenous (IV) vitamin C alleviates a number of cancer- and chemotherapy-related symptoms, such as fatigue, insomnia, loss of appetite, nausea, and pain. Improvements in physical, role, cognitive, emotional, and social functioning, as well as an improvement in overall health, were also observed."[71]

CHAPTER 6

THE TESTOSTERONE FACTOR

Darrel, a 59-year-old firefighter, came to my clinic for the treatment of fatigue, low libido, and loss of muscle mass. Lab testing revealed severe testosterone deficiency. After two months of testosterone replacement, his symptoms were noticeably improved.

◆ ◆ ◆

In Chapter 2 I reviewed the strong connection between prostate enlargement and hormone balance. You learned that testosterone itself is not the culprit but that its metabolite dihydrotestosterone (DHT), an even more potent hormone, can be problematic for the prostate. Furthermore, the class of hormones known as estrogens can cause issues with prostate growth. You also learned in Chapter 5 that these hormones can cause problems for prostate growth, and they can cause problems for prostate cancer as well. In this chapter, you will learn in more depth how to identify and balance your testosterone and estrogen levels for optimal health and vitality.

Many men with prostate problems also suffer from deficiencies and imbalances in testosterone and other male-related hormones. For example, low testosterone affects almost 40 percent of men aged 45 and older![1] Testosterone deficiency can cause fatigue, weight gain, loss of muscle mass, low libido, depression, impotence, and many other symptoms. A testosterone deficiency is even known to be a risk factor for early death.

Other hormones, such as estrogen and dihydrotestosterone, may be elevated in men, contributing to prostate problems such as BPH and prostate cancer. Also, the number of men in America with low libido and erectile dysfunction is quite high, with as many as 30 million men affected by erectile dysfunction.[2] Why just focus on your prostate when great overall health requires proper functioning in all the systems of the body, including testosterone and hormone balance! However, testosterone is a unique hormone that plays a major role in men's health, so it's important to examine all the functions it has in your body. You will see it affects many systems of the body that range from the brain to the heart, muscles and bones, skin, mood and libido, and erectile function.

UNDERSTANDING YOUR TESTOSTERONE LEVELS

Testosterone deficiency negatively affects a man's quality of life and is a known risk factor for early death.[3] Testosterone levels are at their highest by early adulthood and then decrease by 1 to 2 percent a year beginning in the 40s.[4]

The time when testosterone levels drop in middle-aged men is often colloquially referred to as *male menopause.*[5] Another term you might hear is *andropause*, which can be defined as "a syndrome associated with a decrease in sexual satisfaction or a decline in a feeling of general well-being with low levels of testosterone in [an] older man."[6] And lastly, the terms *hypogonadism* and *testicular hypofunction* refer to little or no hormone being produced by the testes.[7]

Deficient levels of testosterone have wide-ranging effects since this hormone acts on almost every tissue in the body.[8] Testosterone has effects on the brain, skin, bones, and heart and impacts erectile function, fat metabolism, muscle growth, bone density, energy production, lipid levels, insulin balance, and much more.

Testosterone deficiency in men increases the risk of all-cause and cardiovascular mortality.[9] For example, a study done on Californian men aged 51 to 91 found that those with low testosterone levels were 40 percent more likely to die than those with higher testosterone levels.[10] Variables that were taken into account include lipid levels, age, and other factors. The same study found low testosterone levels were associated with death from respiratory and cardiovascular disease.

A study published in the *Archives of Internal Medicine* found that veteran males older than 40 years who had a low testosterone level (20 percent of the men in the study) had an increased mortality rate when various factors were taken into account as compared to men with normal testosterone levels.[11]

Another interesting study that included over 11,000 people aged 40 to 79 found that low testosterone levels were significantly associated with mortality from all causes, including cardiovascular disease and cancer.[12]

Low testosterone in men with type 2 diabetes was shown in research to be associated with an increased risk of death versus normal levels of testosterone in men with the same condition. Especially significant was the risk of cardiovascular mortality.[13]

Population studies have shown an increased risk of mortality for those with respiratory diseases who also have low testosterone. This may be due to the medications prescribed for common respiratory diseases such as COPD (chronic obstructive pulmonary disease). Testosterone replacement for men with COPD and asthma has been shown to improve lean body mass, bone density, and sexual quality of life.[14]

People with kidney disease often have testosterone deficiency. It occurs in approximately 44 percent of men with end-stage renal disease, which compromises the quality of their life. One 10-year study of 1,822 men with kidney disease and low testosterone found these men had a more than twofold increase in all-cause mortality.[15]

Common signs and symptoms of testosterone deficiency include reduced energy, reduced endurance, diminished work and/or physical performance, fatigue, depression, reduced sex drive, changes in erectile function (ED), impaired memory, irritability, insomnia, reduced muscle bulk and strength, and increased body fat.[16] Additional possible signs and symptoms of testosterone deficiency include visual changes, anosmia (loss of smell), incomplete or delayed sexual development, loss of body (axillary and pubic) hair, very small testes, breast discomfort, gynecomastia (abnormal swelling of male breast tissue), low sperm count, height loss, low-trauma fractures, low bone mineral density, hot flashes, and sweats.[17]

Conditions associated with testosterone deficiency include unexplained anemia, bone density loss, HIV, diabetes, infertility, and pituitary disorders.[18]

If you experience many of these symptoms or conditions, you'll want to ask your doctor about testosterone testing.

THE SYNTHESIS OF TESTOSTERONE

In the testes, testosterone is produced from the building blocks of cholesterol and acetate (a type of acetic acid). Testosterone production by the testes is regulated by what is known as the hypothalamic-pituitary-gonadal axis (HPG axis). This axis involves messaging from the hypothalamus (an area of the brain) that releases the hormonal messenger gonadotropin-releasing hormone (GnRH). The release of GnRH stimulates the anterior pituitary gland to secrete the hormones luteinizing hormone (LH) and follicle-stimulating hormone (FSH). LH stimulates specialized cells in the testes known as Leydig cells to produce testosterone, whereas FSH stimulates specialized cells in the testes known as Sertoli cells to produce sperm. The hypothalamus secretes GnRH throughout the day in a cyclical fashion, which in turn stimulates the pituitary release of LH and FSH. When testosterone is secreted by the testes and circulating in the bloodstream, specialized receptors in the hypothalamus "sense" the testosterone, which results in an automatic negative feedback action and decreased secretion of GnRH. Estrogen (estradiol) is a metabolite of testosterone and also suppresses GnRH production at the hypothalamus. As a result, LH is inhibited, which results in the testes decreasing their production and release of testosterone. Conversely, if too little testosterone is "sensed" by the hypothalamus, then it responds by secreting GnRH, triggering a corresponding release of LH by the pituitary gland and therefore increased testosterone secretion by the testes.

Most testosterone is bound to carrier molecules. The two main carriers include sex hormone–binding globulin (SHBG) and albumin. Cortisol-binding globulin also acts as a carrier to a lesser degree. The amount of testosterone that is available for activity in the cells is known as "free" or "unbound." Only 2 to 4 percent of circulating testosterone is free or unbound.[19] Total testosterone is the sum of the bound and unbound testosterone in circulation. One other term used in the medical literature is *bioavailable testosterone*, which refers to free and albumin-bound testosterone together. Albumin-bound testosterone dissociates readily and is available to diffuse into tissues, and this is why it is considered bioavailable.

Small amounts of testosterone are also produced from the precursor hormone dehydroepiandrosterone (DHEA). Also, testosterone is converted into the more potent metabolite dihydrotestosterone (DHT) by the enzyme 5-alpha-reductase in the testes, epididymis, prostate, and hair follicles.[20] In addition, testosterone is converted into estrogen by an enzyme known as aromatase, which is located in the liver, nerve, bone, and fat cells.[21] Interestingly, estrogen is important for the maturation of sperm and libido maintenance.[22]

Free testosterone and the metabolites of testosterone such as estrogen (estradiol) and DHT act on cell receptors. DHT is two and a half to three times more potent than testosterone.[23]

Circulating testosterone and DHT are broken down (catabolized) by enzymes in the liver into metabolites that are excreted in the urine.[24]

At the cellular level, testosterone and its metabolite DHT bind to cell receptors known as androgen receptors. This binding to cell receptors causes a cascade of activities that ultimately ends in the hormones interacting with DNA and causing gene transcription (copying of DNA information to RNA) and gene translation (protein synthesis), which is where the effects on tissues take place.[25]

CAUSES OF TESTOSTERONE DEFICIENCY

There are two general categories for the causes of testosterone deficiency. The first is the inability of the testicles to produce testosterone, often referred to as primary hypogonadism. There can be many reasons for this, and often the cause is unknown. Examples would include the following:[26]

- genetic causes
- chemotherapy
- radiation therapy
- removal of testicles (due to reasons such as cancer)
- testicle resistance to the messaging hormone LH

The second cause is dysfunctional external factors that influence the testicles. Examples include the following:[27]

- hyperprolactinemia (excess production of the hormone prolactin by the pituitary gland, usually due to a benign tumor but sometimes from medications)
- severe obesity
- iron overload
- use of certain medications such as opioids, glucocorticoids, ketoconazole, cimetidine, spironolactone, certain antidepressants, chemotherapy drugs, and cholesterol-lowering statin drugs[28]

- anabolic steroid abuse

- tumors of the hypothalamus or pituitary

- head trauma

- pituitary surgery or radiation

- endocrine-disrupting chemicals (see the examples in the next section)

It is also important to note that testosterone levels can be affected by acute illness, nutritional deficiency or alcoholism, eating disorders, sleep disorders (including obstructive sleep apnea), and excessive exercise.[29]

Environmental Concerns for Testosterone Imbalance

As previously listed, endocrine-disrupting chemicals (EDCs) are problematic for the proper functioning of the hormone system. These chemicals are found in commonly used products such as water bottles, plastics, cosmetics, canned food, fertilizers, toothpastes, clothes, soaps, paper, textiles, carpets, utensils, deodorants, bedding, and from other items that end up in the body.[30] It is recognized that EDCs interfere with the synthesis and action of sex hormones such as testosterone.[31] There is a correlation between an increase in several EDCs and declining sperm count and testosterone levels.[32] Be mindful of the following common toxins:

- *Phthalates*, which are used in plastics, have been found in the urine of 75 percent of Americans.[33] Phthalates disrupt testosterone production by interfering with the metabolism of cholesterol in the Leydig cells of the testes.[34] Cholesterol is required to synthesize testosterone.

- *Bisphenol A (BPA)* is a plasticizer found in the urine of most Americans. BPA has been shown to disrupt testosterone synthesis by blocking LH receptors on Leydig cells.[35]

- *Dioxins* and *PCB* are EDCs that disrupt the hypothalamic-pituitary-thyroid axis, which regulates steroid production, thus decreasing testosterone.[36] Dioxins are by-products of industrial processes such as smelting, chlorine bleaching of paper pulp, and the manufacturing of some pesticides and herbicides. Most dioxins enter the body through the food chain, especially meat and dairy products, fish, and shellfish. They accumulate in the fat tissues of humans and other animals.

- *Insecticides* are commonly found in the urine of men. Research has shown that certain pesticides are associated with reduced testosterone levels.[37] A study in the *International Journal of Reproduction, Contraception, Obstetrics and Gynecology* revealed that pesticides and insecticides significantly decrease serum testosterone and sperm levels.[38]

- *Toxic metals* are also a concern for testosterone deficiency. For example, organic mercury is a common contaminant in our environment. Sources include fossil fuel emissions, the burning of medical waste, dental amalgams, vaccines, and incandescent lights. The major form is methylmercury, which accumulates

in fish and is consumed by humans. Research
has demonstrated that mercury can alter
the messaging system of the hypothalamic-
pituitary-gonadal axis and affect reproductive
function and circulating testosterone levels.[39]

The avoidance of endocrine disruptors is important. This can be accomplished through ingesting purified water and organic foods and using "clean" cosmetics and personal care items. Also, regular detoxification
support through exercise, sauna therapy, and detoxifying
nutraceuticals is recommended. (Please see Chapter 9 for
more details.)

TESTING FOR
TESTOSTERONE DEFICIENCY

If you have any of the signs and symptoms of testosterone deficiency, please talk to your integrative care provider
about testing.

The primary test for testosterone deficiency is total
testosterone. There is not a consensus as to what precise
range indicates a deficient blood level of total testosterone.
Laboratories differ in their testosterone reference ranges,
although they normally range from 250 ng/dL to 400 ng/
dL and up to 1000 to 1100 ng/dL. The American Urological
Association states that a total testosterone level below 300
ng/dL is a reasonable cutoff for healthy testosterone. The
Endocrine Society notes that the lower limit for normal
total testosterone for healthy, nonobese young men by labs
that are certified by the Centers for Disease Control (CDC)
is 264 ng/dL (9.2 nmol/L). The International Society for

Sexual Medicine (ISSM) uses a total testosterone of less than 350 ng/dL (12 nmol) as a cutoff point, although it is reasonable to offer testosterone therapy to symptomatic patients with levels above 350 ng/dL.[40]

Testosterone deficiency should be diagnosed with two separate total testosterone measurements in the early morning (8 or 9 A.M.). This is because serum testosterone levels vary significantly due to normal hormonal rhythms of the endocrine system and are highest in the early morning.[41]

It's important to note that approximately 30 percent of men who have an initial low testosterone level will have a normal level with repeat measurement.[42] You can have the repeated test any other day of the week in the morning.

If the total testosterone level is low to normal or borderline, especially in obese or older men, then sex hormone–binding globulin (SHBG) and free testosterone should be tested or calculated.

The Endocrine Society recommends against routine screening of men for testosterone deficiency.[43] I think this is a mistake, since it is better to find a health problem early while the root cause(s) can still be potentially addressed.

Common Tests Used for Diagnosing Testosterone Deficiency

While testosterone levels can be tested through saliva and urine, blood total testosterone is the standard test. Serum total testosterone, specifically, is the primary test used to diagnose testosterone deficiency. As mentioned above, it is preferably administered in the early morning (8 to 9 A.M.).

However, I recommend comprehensive hormone testing that goes beyond total testosterone. There are two reasons for this. First, additional tests can help pinpoint why you have testosterone deficiency. Second, your hormones work like an orchestra. So if additional hormones are deficient, then addressing them helps you feel better and improves your overall hormone communication and balance.

For more comprehensive testing beyond testosterone levels, your doctor should order blood work to measure the following:

- *Free Testosterone:* This test is important if sex hormone–binding globulin is abnormal (best is a lab that uses equilibrium dialysis or use as a calculation).

- *Luteinizing Hormone (LH):* This helps to determine if the testosterone deficiency is caused by a problem with the hypothalamus or pituitary gland. Low or low/normal levels may require further investigation.

- *Prolactin:* This is another pituitary hormone. An elevated level may suggest a pituitary tumor that is causing a pituitary messaging problem to the testes. Further evaluation, such as a pituitary MRI, would be indicated in elevated prolactin levels.

- *Estradiol:* A baseline level is good to establish to compare future levels if on testosterone therapy. Also, elevated baseline levels in men who are deficient in testosterone and have breast discomfort or gynecomastia (breast enlargement) indicate the need for referral to a specialist for evaluation.

- *PSA:* A baseline test is done to screen for prostate abnormalities and to compare the baseline to future repeat testing.

- *Sex Hormone–Binding Globulin (SHBG):* This protein binds and transports testosterone and estradiol. If levels are high, then free testosterone levels will be lower.

- *Cortisol:* This is an adrenal stress hormone that, when high, can interfere with testosterone metabolism. Saliva testing is the preferred method.

- *DHEA:* This is an adrenal stress hormone that has similar effects to testosterone and is also a precursor to testosterone.

- *Pregnenolone:* This is another adrenal stress hormone.

- *IGF1:* This marker reflects growth hormone activity.

- *Complete Blood Count (CBC):* Red blood cells are monitored to make sure they are not increasing.

- *Complete Metabolic Panel (CMP):* This test measures liver and kidney function, electrolytes, and glucose.

- *Ferritin:* This indicates iron stores.

- *Vitamin D:* A deficiency in vitamin D is linked to lower testosterone levels.

- *Vitamin B12:* This vitamin is important for proper energy levels.

- *Hemoglobin A1C:* This is used in long-term blood glucose regulation.

- *Fasting Insulin:* This is a marker for insulin resistance that is associated with lower testosterone.

- *Comprehensive Cardiovascular Profile:* This test should include not only lipids but also lipoproteins and inflammation markers (e.g., total cholesterol, HDL cholesterol, triglycerides, non-HDL and calculated components, lipoprotein fractionation, ion mobility, apolipoprotein B, lipoprotein(a), hs-CRP, Lp-PLA2 activity, oxidized LDL, fibrinogen, and homocysteine).

The following tests should also be ordered:

- *Urinalysis:* This test assesses kidney function.

- *Bone Density (DEXA):* This scan rules out osteoporosis in men. While this test is not often ordered by doctors, the fact is that up to 25 percent of men over age 50 will break a bone due to osteoporosis.[44]

PROTOCOL FOR TESTOSTERONE DEFICIENCY

If you have a diagnosis of testosterone deficiency or suboptimal testosterone levels, then the following diet and supplements can be helpful. This nonpharmaceutical protocol can be followed for three months, after which levels should be rechecked. For men that require testosterone replacement based on the diagnosis of a doctor, see the hormone replacement section and consult with a doctor knowledgeable in bioidentical hormone replacement, as it requires a prescription and monitoring.

Diet and Lifestyle

The Western diet is associated with lower testosterone levels in men. A study in the journal *Nutrients* demonstrated that the Standard American Diet (SAD) is significantly associated with low total testosterone levels and an unhealthy body composition (decreased skeletal muscle mass and increased visceral fat mass). More specifically, this study found that dietary patterns "characterized by high-frequency consumption of bread and pastries, dairy products, and desserts, eating out, and low intake frequency of homemade foods, noodles, and dark green vegetables" were significantly associated with low testosterone.[45]

High consumption of refined carbohydrates is associated with conditions known to be related to low testosterone levels, including obesity, metabolic syndrome, nonalcoholic fatty liver disease, and insulin resistance.[46]

Excess alcohol intake is also associated with low testosterone.

A modified Mediterranean diet is a good choice for men with low testosterone. A plethora of studies show the traditional Mediterranean diet reduces the risks of major diseases. The traditional diet revolves around vegetables, fruits, seafood, poultry, beans, herbs and spices, olive oil, nuts, moderate dairy, and limited red meat. See Chapter 8 and the Appendix for meal-planning tips.

Proper Sleep

Treating sleep disorders is an important step toward promoting a balanced hormonal system. It is also vital to get adequate sleep each evening. On the other hand, testosterone deficiency may contribute to some men's difficulties getting healthy sleep. Therefore, testosterone replacement, along with weight management, helps some men with their sleep quality.[47]

Exercise

Resistance training is typically recommended for improving testosterone levels in men. However, a study of 87 men with erectile dysfunction who followed aerobic exercise with stationary cycling had a better increase of testosterone than those who performed strengthening exercises. The total amount of exercise may be more important than the type of exercise.[48]

Research has demonstrated that the combination of testosterone replacement and exercise improves testosterone deficiency symptoms better than testosterone replacement alone. The type of exercise in these studies was mainly resistance strengthening exercises.[49]

SUPPLEMENTS FOR TESTOSTERONE DEFICIENCY

Nutritional supplements, especially specific herbal extracts, are an excellent choice for men with mildly low or suboptimal testosterone levels. They are also a great choice for men with normal total testosterone levels but low or suboptimal free testosterone levels. The following are supplements with good research demonstrating their ability to increase male testosterone levels.

Ashwagandha

Ashwagandha (*Withania somnifera*) is used in Ayurvedic medicine as a "rejuvenator" to promote health and longevity, combat the effects of aging, and create a sense of well-being.[50] Ashwagandha also possesses anti-inflammatory, antistress, and antioxidant properties.[51] This revered herb has been shown in published clinical research to reduce fatigue, anxiety, irritability, inability to concentrate, and forgetfulness.[52] And ashwagandha has a history of use in Ayurvedic medicine to treat male sexual dysfunction and infertility and to act as an aphrodisiac.[53]

Ashwagandha is accepted as an herbal adaptogen.[54] The European Medicines Agency (EMA) defines herbal adaptogens as follows:

> Adaptogenic substances are stated to have the capacity to normalize body functions and strengthen systems compromised by stress. They are reported to have a protective effect on health against a wide variety of environmental assaults and emotional conditions.[55]

Ashwagandha has a balancing effect on the hormonal system of the body. It has been shown in human studies to increase serum testosterone levels and decrease serum cortisol.[56] Ashwagandha contains several active components that likely account for its effects on the hypothalamic-pituitary-adrenal axis (HPA). These include saponins and alkaloids, steroidal lactones (withanolides, withaferins), amino acids, and neurotransmitters.[57]

Ashwagandha extract has been shown to significantly increase testosterone levels compared to placebo in men.[58] In this eight-week, randomized, prospective, placebo-controlled, double-blind study, 57 men ages 18 to 50 with little experience in resistance training were given ashwagandha extract (300 mg) or a placebo twice daily. Baseline measurements were taken, and then the men followed a resistance training program. Their measurements were retaken at the end of the eight weeks. Researchers found the men taking ashwagandha extract had significantly increased testosterone levels (96.19 ng/dL) compared to those taking a placebo (18.0 ng/dL). The men taking ashwagandha extract also had a significantly greater increase in muscle strength as measured with bench press and leg extension exercises, increased muscle size of the arms and chest, greater decreases in body fat percentage (3.5 percent compared to 1.5 percent for placebo), and decreased exercise-induced muscle damage (as measured by serum creatine kinase level). None of the participants experienced adverse effects.

A study published in *Evidence-Based Complementary and Alternative Medicine* looked at the effect of ashwagandha extract on hormone levels (including testosterone) and the sperm-producing (spermatogenic) activity of 46 men with low sperm count (oligospermic). In the study, 46 males were randomized to receive either ashwagandha extract (675 mg per day) or placebo. Serum hormone levels (testosterone and LH) were tested at the beginning and end of the 90-day study. Serum testosterone increased significantly, by 17 percent, and LH (which stimulates testes production of testosterone) increased by 34 percent as compared to baseline. Participants taking a placebo did not have an increase in testosterone levels.[59]

Another study published in the *American Journal of Men's Health* involved overweight men aged 40 to 70 who experienced fatigue. This 16-week, randomized, double-blind, placebo-controlled crossover study compared the effects of ashwagandha extract (600 mg) to placebo. Although energy levels were not significantly improved in the men taking ashwagandha, they saw a significant increase in testosterone (15 percent) and DHEA-S (18 percent) salivary levels compared to placebo. There was no statistically significant difference in salivary cortisol or estradiol levels compared to placebo.[60]

Recommendation: 600 to 675 mg daily of a standardized extract, as recommended by published studies

Safety: Ashwagandha is well tolerated.

Eurycoma longifolia

Eurycoma longifolia, also known as tongkat ali, is recognized in countries such as Malaysia, Thailand, and Indonesia as an herbal medicine to support male sexual disorders and infertility. The roots of this plant are often referred to as "Malaysian ginseng." The government of Malaysia has invested in the scientific research of *Eurycoma longifolia* and has taken out a patent along with the Massachusetts Institute of Technology for a well-studied water extract from the root.[61] This extract is available as a dietary supplement in the United States.

Eurycoma longifolia has been shown to improve erectile function, libido, and male sexual well-being, as well as stimulate the synthesis of testosterone.[62]

Eurycoma longifolia has been shown to increase both total testosterone (bound form in the blood) and free testosterone (unbound form).[63] In a study published in the *Journal of the International Society of Sports Nutrition*, researchers looked at the effects of 200 mg of *Eurycoma longifolia* extract on people who were "moderately stressed." Compared to placebo, those taking the extract had a significant increase in testosterone (37 percent) and a significant decrease in cortisol (16 percent). Furthermore, those taking the extract had significant improvements in tension, anger, and confusion.[64]

In a five-week study of physically active male and female seniors (ages 57 to 72), supplementation with *Eurycoma longifolia* extract (400 mg daily) was shown to significantly increase total and free testosterone concentrations and muscular force in men and women. Handgrip strength measures improved as a reflection of an increase in muscle force. No side effects were noted for those supplementing *Eurycoma longifolia* extract.[65]

The active substance in *Eurycoma longifolia* that works to improve testosterone levels is unknown. However, the extract from this plant has chains of amino acids (polypeptides) that activate the liver enzyme CYP17 to increase the production of DHEA and androstenedione.[66] Furthermore, the cortisol-lowering effects of *Eurycoma longifolia* may benefit the levels of free testosterone.

Recommendation: 200 to 400 mg daily of an extract

Safety: *Eurycoma longifolia* has been shown in a review of studies to be safe based on no significant changes in liver or kidney function tests.[67]

Additional Nutrients to Support Testosterone Production

Deficiencies in the following nutrients can lead to low testosterone levels. I recommend supplementing with the following:

- *Zinc:* Zinc deficiency is common throughout the world, including the United States. The mineral zinc is very important for male sexual function and is found in high concentrations in the testes, prostate, and semen.[68] It is also involved in the synthesis of testosterone, and deficiency is associated with low testosterone in men. Zinc supplementation is more likely to help men with testosterone deficiency who have a zinc deficiency. A study of zinc supplementation in healthy, elderly men with mild zinc deficiency observed that supplementation doubled their serum testosterone levels in six months.[69]

  Recommendation: A typical supplemental dose is 25 to 50 mg daily with a meal.

- *Vitamin D:* Studies are mixed as to whether vitamin D deficiency is a causative factor in testosterone deficiency. Serum vitamin D testing can easily identify if a male has a vitamin D deficiency that requires treatment.

  Recommendation: A typical supplemental dose is 2000 to 5000 IU daily with a meal.

- *Magnesium:* Magnesium supplementation has been shown to increase free and total testosterone levels in young male athletes as well as healthy sedentary subjects.[70]
  Recommendation: A typical supplemental dose is 250 to 500 mg daily.

TESTOSTERONE REPLACEMENT

Testosterone replacement is indicated for men who have diagnosed testosterone deficiency. The American Urological Association and the Endocrine Society have published guidelines on the evaluation and management of testosterone deficiency. I summarized their recommendations earlier in this chapter, pages 122 and 123.[71]

Testosterone replacement in men with a diagnosed deficiency has been shown to

- improve sexual function (significantly improving libido, erectile function, and sexual activity in men with low libido)

- improve well-being and depressive symptoms (except in men with clinical depression)

- increase bone density and strength

- improve body composition, muscle strength, and physical function—testosterone therapy in healthy men with testosterone deficiency reduces the whole-body, intra-abdominal, and intermuscular fat[72]

Cautions for Testosterone Replacement

Testosterone replacement is not typically recommended for men who are planning to have children, as it can suppress sperm production. It is also not recommended for men who have breast or prostate cancer, prostate nodules or hardness (induration) that has not been evaluated by a urologist, elevated PSA levels (unless prostate problems such as prostate cancer have been ruled out), elevated hematocrit (excess red blood cells), untreated severe obstructive sleep apnea, severe LUTS, uncontrolled heart failure, or thrombophilia, or who have experienced a heart attack or stroke in the past six months.[73]

A 2019 article in the *Journal of Clinical Medicine* summarizes the safety of testosterone replacement therapy. The authors note that testosterone replacement in testosterone-deficient older men did not significantly increase the rate of prostate cancer compared to those who received a placebo.[74]

The Endogenous Hormones and Prostate Cancer Collaborative Group analyzed 95 percent of worldwide published data on the relationship between serum testosterone and prostate cancer.[75] The analysis included 18 prospective trials of 3,886 men with prostate cancer and 6,439 controls. They found no associations between prostate cancer and serum levels of free and total testosterone.

There has been a paradigm shift in the use of testosterone replacement for men with a history of prostate cancer. Testosterone replacement is becoming more common in men with a history of cured prostate cancer who had a prostatectomy with favorable pathology (e.g., negative margins, no signs of metastasis, and undetectable PSA).[76] Also, men with a history of radiation therapy for prostate cancer (with or without androgen deprivation therapy) who are treated with testosterone therapy do not tend to experience recurrence or progression of prostate cancer and tend to experience a decline in PSA or have nonsignificant changes in PSA.[77]

Testosterone replacement therapy is becoming an accepted option for selected men with a history of prostate cancer who have no evidence of disease recurrence as well as for men with low-risk prostate cancer under active surveillance.[78]

Updated research is more optimistic regarding the cardiovascular risk of testosterone therapy. Researchers analyzed data of almost 20,000 men who received testosterone therapy for five years (from 2009 to 2014). They found the risk for a heart attack was sevenfold lower and the risk for stroke nine times lower compared with samples from the general population. Further, there was no evidence of worsening of preexisting heart attack or stroke in patients treated with testosterone. Their analysis found that testosterone therapy in men is not associated with an increased risk for heart attack or stroke, and it may even be cardioprotective![79]

Where to Obtain Bioidentical Hormones

Bioidentical testosterone and other bioidentical hormones are available through prescription from your doctor. Once you have a prescription, it's up to you where you obtain your hormones. However, it's important to note that conventional pharmacies carry only expensive, trade name hormones. I recommend that you seek out compounding pharmacies. These specialized pharmacies can formulate natural hormones that meet the specific needs of the patient.

Most cities have compounding pharmacies. Due to what I believe to be the influence of America's pharmaceutical giants, there has been a smear campaign against compounding pharmacies. The reason: the cost of bioidentical hormones through a compounding pharmacy is very low relative to the big, trade name hormones available through regular pharmacies. Big Pharma is not happy that an effective, much lower-cost product is available to consumers. The claim by Big Pharma and its allies is that compounded drugs are not regulated by the FDA. However, the suppliers that compounding pharmacies get their ingredients from are registered and inspected by the FDA. Also, all pharmacists and pharmacies are licensed and regulated strictly by state boards of pharmacy. And in reality, the FDA has authority over some aspects of compounded medications at the federal level.[80]

HORMONE ORCHESTRA

Your many hormones work in conjunction with one another like musicians in an orchestra. This is why I test the other major hormones such as thyroid, DHEA, pregnenolone, and several others and balance or replace them for the optimal functioning of the whole hormonal system.

There are certain common hormonal issues that may come up with testosterone replacement.

- *For elevated estrogen levels:* If estrogen (estradiol and estrone) levels are elevated, then the use of supplemental zinc (100 mg with 2 mg of copper) or ground flaxseed (1 to 2 tablespoons), broccoli extract (indole-3-carbinol 200 to 400 mg or diindolylmethane

100 to 200 mg), chrysin (250 mg), or certain
Chinese herbal formulas can help lower
levels by inhibiting the enzyme aromatase,
which converts testosterone into estrogen.
For more severe cases, the estrogen-blocking
medication anastrozole (0.5 mg twice weekly)
may be used. The prescribing doctor can
lower the testosterone dose as well.

- *For elevated DHT levels:* If dihydrotestosterone
  (DHT) levels are elevated, then the use
  of transdermal progesterone (20 mg) can
  be helpful.

When and How to Use Testosterone Replacement

There are several ways to administer bioidentical testosterone, including topical gels and creams, patches, buccal tablets (oral), sublingual drops, intramuscular (IM) injections, and pellet implants. Common starting doses for transdermal creams and gels are 50 to 100 mg daily; for IM injections, 100 mg once weekly. Testosterone is not given as an oral capsule or tablet due to the risk of liver toxicity when ingested in this way. (Buccal tablets are taken orally but not swallowed—they dissolve in the mucosa of the mouth, so they go directly into the bloodstream.)

For younger males with low testosterone, it is preferable to use the herbal and nutritional supplements combined with diet and lifestyle changes. If these are not effective, then medications that enhance the body's production of testosterone and maintain fertility, such as clomiphene citrate (50 mg three times weekly) and human chorionic gonadotropin (HCG), are preferred. HCG is the preferred treatment in younger men.

Human chorionic gonadotropin can also be used for men on testosterone replacement if there is a decrease in testicular size (atrophy). A typical regimen is 1000 units injected twice weekly, with breaks in use every two months.

In a study of 282 men with low testosterone, the men were randomized to receive one of three treatments: clomiphene citrate 50 mg daily, HCG injections 5000 IU twice weekly, or a combination of both therapies. Researchers found that all three treatments were equally effective in increasing testosterone levels.[81]

Monitoring Testosterone Replacement

I normally repeat blood work—including a CBC (to see if red blood cells are increasing, a process known as erythrocytosis), metabolic panel (to monitor liver and kidney function), total testosterone, estradiol, and PSA—after six to eight weeks of testosterone supplementation. If levels are normal and the patient's signs and symptoms are progressing in a positive direciton, then lab testing is repeated every four to six months. A prostate examination with a digital rectal exam should be completed by a doctor yearly. If the PSA increases more than 1.4 ng/mL with the use of testosterone replacement, the Endocrine Society recommends a referral to a urologist.

The preferred timing of phlebotomy (blood draw) is in the morning before the application of a testosterone gel or cream. If a patient is being administered the injectable form of testosterone, then phlebotomy is done midway between injections.

As you have read, testosterone is a critically important hormone for men's health. It should be checked for imbalances and supported through diet, lifestyle, supplements, and the proper use of testosterone replacement, if needed.

CHAPTER 7

ERASING ERECTILE DYSFUNCTION AND BOOSTING LIBIDO

Todd, a 62-year-old accountant, had a great relationship with his wife and decent health aside from being slightly over-weight. However, he could not understand why his libido was low and erectile dysfunction was becoming more problematic year after year. Testing showed testosterone deficiency as well as the beginning of atherosclerosis (hardening of the arteries). A major change in his diet and exercise program, testosterone replacement, and nutritional supplements to improve circula-tion were very helpful in improving his symptoms.

◆ ◆ ◆

Low libido and erectile dysfunction (ED) are common problems that can be connected to testosterone deficiency, as well as other causes. For example, about 5 percent of men overall and 41 percent of men between the ages of 66 and 74 have decreased libido.[1] As many as 30 million men have experienced problems with ED.[2] In this chapter, I will discuss these two issues, their causes, and their inte-grative solutions.

ERECTILE DYSFUNCTION

Erectile dysfunction refers to the inability to get or keep an erection for sexual intercourse. What once was thought to be a psychological problem has been shown in research to be much more often a physical problem. However, once a physical issue is causing ED, then psychological factors often come into play as well—making the problem worse.

ED as a symptom should be a red flag to your doctor to look for underlying health problems, such as cardiovascular disease. Diseases of the cardiovascular system account for almost 50 percent of all ED cases.[3] This includes diseases such as atherosclerosis (hardening of the arteries), peripheral vascular disease, heart attack, and high blood pressure.[4]

Research has shown that men with ED have a higher risk of death, irrespective of their testosterone levels (which can also boost death risk if low). A large observational study investigated age-related hormonal changes and general health outcomes in 1,913 elderly men.[5] The relationship between testosterone levels and sexual function was measured at the beginning of the study and again for men who were alive 12 years later. Researchers found that in men with normal testosterone levels with the presence of sexual symptoms, especially ED, there was a 51 percent increased risk of death compared with men without sexual symptoms. Men who had ED, poor morning erections, and low libido had a 1.8 times higher mortality rate compared to men with no sexual symptoms. Also, in men who had ED and no other symptoms, the risk of dying was 1.4 times higher than in men who did not have ED.

Causes of ED

There are many diseases that may cause ED, including diabetes, high blood pressure, high cholesterol, coronary artery disease, neurological diseases, hormone imbalances, BPH, sleep apnea, chronic obstructive pulmonary disease (COPD), and depression.[6] Following is a summary of the different categories of diseases associated with ED:[7]

- *Blood vessel–related (vascular) diseases:* atherosclerosis, peripheral vascular disease, myocardial infarction, arterial hypertension, vascular injury from radiation therapy, vascular injury from prostate cancer treatment, blood vessel and nerve trauma (e.g., from long-distance bicycle riding)

- *Systemic diseases:* diabetes mellitus, scleroderma, renal failure, liver cirrhosis, idiopathic hemochromatosis, cancer and cancer treatment, dyslipidemia, hypertension

- *Nerve-related (neurological) diseases:* epilepsy, stroke, multiple sclerosis, Guillain-Barré syndrome, Alzheimer's disease, trauma

- *Respiratory diseases:* COPD, sleep apnea

- *Hormone (endocrine) diseases:* hyperthyroidism, hypothyroidism, hypogonadism, diabetes

- *Penile diseases:* Peyronie's disease (bent penis caused by scar tissue), epispadias (birth defect with malformation of penis), priapism (prolonged erection)

- *Psychiatric diseases:* depression, widower's syndrome, performance anxiety, post-traumatic stress disorder

- *Nutritional imbalances:* malnutrition, zinc deficiency

- *Blood (hematological) diseases:* sickle cell anemia, leukemia

- *Surgical procedures:* brain and spinal cord procedures, retroperitoneal or pelvic lymph node dissection, aortoiliac or aortofemoral bypass, abdominoperineal resection, proctocolectomy, transurethral resection of the prostate, radical prostatectomy, cryosurgery of the prostate, cystectomy

- *Trauma:* injuries to the pelvic blood vessels or nerves

- *Medications:* antidepressants, antipsychotics, antiulcer agents (e.g., cimetidine), 5-alpha-reductase inhibitors (e.g., finasteride and dutasteride), blood pressure–lowering drugs, cholesterol-lowering agents, methadone, opioids, testosterone abuse

- *Smoking:* Research has shown that male smokers with ED who stop smoking had significantly better ED status compared to current smokers after one year of follow-up.[8]

- *Pornography overconsumption:* According to the International Society for Sexual Medicine, "Sustained pornography use can have some serious effects on a person's relationships, mental health, social and work interactions, and sexual function."[9]

Pharmaceutical Medications for ED

The common class of ED medications are the oral phosphodiesterase type 5 (PDE5) inhibitors, which includes sildenafil (Viagra), vardenafil (Levitra and Staxyn), tadalafil (Cialis), and avanafil (Stendra). The most commonly prescribed ED drug in America is Viagra or its generic version, sildenafil.[10]

These drugs work by inhibiting the PDE5 enzyme. Normally, PDE5 breaks down the cellular messenger known as cGMP. By keeping cGMP around longer, these drugs cause relaxation of the smooth muscle in blood vessels that supply penile blood flow. Only tadalafil (Cialis) is taken on a daily basis for the treatment of both ED and BPH.

INTEGRATIVE SOLUTIONS FOR ED

Regular daily exercise is highly recommended for men with ED. Exercise improves pelvic blood flow and reduces the effects of stress. A longitudinal study found that older adult men who are physically active have less erectile difficulties and increased sexual activity.

Diet is also important for the prevention and treatment of ED. As discussed earlier, good cardiovascular health and blood flow are critical for healthy erectile function.[11] A healthy diet is essential for healthy blood vessels and blood flow.

A review of four clinical trials of men with ED who were consuming the Mediterranean diet found it to be effective in preventing ED and preserving sexual function.[12] Another study of men with ED and metabolic syndrome (elevated blood glucose, excess body fat around the waist, high blood pressure, and abnormal triglyceride or cholesterol levels) found that the Mediterranean diet improved the quality of erections.[13]

Supplements

- *L-arginine* is an amino acid present in dietary proteins and is produced in the kidneys from the amino acid L-citrulline. L-arginine is a precursor to the compound nitric oxide (NO). NO causes smooth muscle relaxation and blood vessel dilation in the penile tissues, which helps erections. Some studies demonstrate that 2800 to 6000 mg of L-arginine daily results in beneficial effects, although it seems to work better when combined with Pycnogenol.[14]

  Recommendation: up to 6000 mg daily (or 1700 mg L-arginine in combination with 120 mg Pycnogenol daily)

  Safety: L-arginine is quite safe. Consult with your doctor before using if you are on medications for blood pressure, angina, blood clot prevention or treatment, or ED.

- *Pycnogenol (pine bark extract)* in combination with L-arginine appears to be more effective than L-arginine alone. Studies show this combination significantly improves erectile function, increases the duration of erections, and decreases the time to achieve erection.[15] In one three-month study of this combination (L-arginine 1700 mg and Pycnogenol 120 mg per day), 92.5 percent of subjects experienced a normal erection.[16]

Recommendation: 120 mg Pycnogenol (in combination with 1700 mg L-arginine) per day

Safety: Pycnogenol is quite safe. Consult with your doctor before using if you are on medication for blood pressure, blood clot prevention or treatment, or ED.

- *L-citrulline* is an amino acid that acts as a precursor to nitric oxide. Research has shown that L-citrulline increases L-arginine blood levels.[17] In a small study of men with mild ED, it was shown to be effective in improving erectile function.[18]

  Recommendation: 500 mg three times daily on an empty stomach

  Safety: L-citrulline is quite safe. Consult with your doctor before using if you are on medication for blood pressure, angina, blood clot prevention or treatment, or ED.

- *Korean red ginseng* was shown in a study published in the *International Journal of Impotence Research* to improve erectile function.[19] A review of seven randomized controlled trials found that Korean red ginseng is effective in the treatment of ED.[20] Ginseng has been shown to increase NO synthesis, which would explain the benefit for ED.[21] Doses used in studies vary from 1800 to 2700 mg daily, with much lower doses, such as 300 mg daily, used when concentrated standardized extracts are administered.

Recommendation: 300 to 900 mg daily

Safety: Consult with your doctor before using if you are on medication for blood pressure, antiandrogen therapy, or blood clot prevention or treatment.

Hormone Therapy

Among aging men, better levels of testosterone and DHEA are associated with fewer problems with ED.[22] Men with low testosterone have a greater prevalence of ED compared to men with normal testosterone levels. Also, several studies have shown that testosterone replacement improves ED for men with low testosterone.[23] See Chapter 6 for more information on testosterone replacement.

Additional Medical Therapies for ED

- *Vacuum devices:* These products draw blood into the penis before sexual activity and have been shown to be effective in 50 to 90 percent of patients in helping maintain an erection for up to 30 minutes.[24] The procedure involves placing a plastic cylinder over the penis. Air is then pumped out, causing a vacuum effect, and then after an erection occurs, a constricting band is placed around the base of the penis.

- *Injection of vasodilators:* Injection-delivered medications that cause vasodilation and erection are available by prescription. This type of approach may be recommended if oral ED medications are ineffective. The procedure involves injecting a medication into the side of the shaft of the penis before sexual activity. Side effects can include bleeding, pain, priapism, and scarring inside the tissue that holds the blood.[25]

  The most common agent used is alprostadil, which was shown in one large study to be effective in 94 percent of men.[26] Today most doctors prescribe a combination of medications in one injection. Trimix is a common formula that contains the vasodilators papaverine hydrochloride, phentolamine, and PGE1 (alprostadil).[27]

- *Shock wave therapy:* There is emerging evidence that low-intensity shock wave therapy is effective for men with ED who do not respond to PDE5 inhibitors.[28] Shock wave therapy uses energy from sound waves that pass through penile tissue and stimulate blood flow. Most patients do not require anesthesia. Treatments last about 15 minutes and are repeated weekly for six weeks.[29] Cleveland Clinic doctors have found success about 62 percent of the time.[30]

LOW LIBIDO

Low libido or low sex drive is common in men, and there are many reasons for it, including aging, chronic illness (e.g., cancer), depression, stress, relationship problems, medications (antidepressants, high blood pressure medications, antihistamines and decongestants, narcotics, chemotherapy drugs), alcohol abuse, insomnia, under- or overexercising, poor body image, and low self-esteem.[31]

The Diagnostic and Statistical Manual of Mental Disorders (DSM-5) recognizes a condition known as male hypoactive sexual desire disorder that essentially refers to a low level of sexual interest and the lack of initiating or responding to sexual intimacy.[32] This persistent lack of interest must cause distress or impairment in the man's life or relationships.[33] With this diagnosis there must be no other medical condition or factor (such as drug abuse or medications) that is causing the low libido.

INTEGRATIVE SOLUTIONS FOR LOW LIBIDO

The best treatment for a man's low libido is to treat the underlying root causes. For example, if the primary problem is high stress levels, along with anxiety and depression, then therapy that focuses on these issues is best. Also, a lot of men will be surprised how much their libidos will improve when they follow a healthy diet, get proper sleep, and exercise regularly. Improving communication and quality time with one's spouse is also important for improving libido.

You may also find the following supplements helpful:

- *Eurycoma longifolia* (tongkat ali) is popular in Malaysia, Thailand, and Indonesia as a plant medicine for the treatment of male sexual disorders. An extract from the root has been shown to improve libido in men.[34]

  Recommendation: 200 to 400 mg daily of an extract

  Safety: *Eurycoma longifolia* has been shown in a review of studies to be safe based on no significant changes in liver or kidney function tests.[35]

- Maca (*Lepidium meyenii*) has been traditionally used in Peru for its aphrodisiac effects. In a 12-week, double-blind, placebo-controlled, randomized, parallel trial, men aged 21 to 56 received 1500 mg of maca, 3000 mg of maca, or a placebo. Maca was shown to improve sexual desire at 8 and 12 weeks of treatment.[36]

  Recommendation: 1500 to 3000 mg daily

  Safety: Maca has been shown to be very safe.

If you suffer from anxiety, then consider the following in addition to counseling and lifestyle changes:

- *GABA (gamma-aminobutyric acid):* This is an amino acid that is available as a supplement. It activates GABA receptors in the parasympathetic nervous system, which causes a relaxation effect.

Recommendation: 100 to 200 mg two to three times daily on an empty stomach

Safety: GABA is quite safe. Do not mix with medications that act on GABA receptors without your doctor's consent.

If anxiety and/or depression is problematic, then consider this supplement:

- *5-HTP (5-Hydroxytryptophan):* This is a building block of the neurotransmitter serotonin.

  Recommendation: 100 mg three times daily on an empty stomach

  Safety: Digestive upset may occur. Do not take in conjunction with antidepressants without your doctor's consent.

Hormone Therapy

The use of bioidentical dehydroepiandrosterone and testosterone can be helpful for low libido. There are several studies demonstrating that testosterone replacement in men with testosterone deficiency results in the significant improvement of libido in men.[37] Testosterone replacement was also shown to improve sexual desire in aging men with low-normal testosterone levels.[38] Testing and treatment with an integrative doctor is recommended. See Chapter 6 for more information.

CHAPTER 8

SUPERNUTRITION FOR THE PROSTATE

Do not underestimate the power that diet has in preventing and treating prostate conditions. The foods you eat can promote healthy or unhealthy prostate cells.

Several studies have demonstrated that the right foods can dramatically reduce the risks of prostate cancer, prostatitis, erectile dysfunction, and BPH. A recent review of 35 articles on the effect of diet on BPH, LUTS, and ED found that food is an important factor affecting the risk of developing BPH and ED.[1] Furthermore, many positive studies show that diet affects prostate cancer risk. These studies are reviewed in each of the chapters devoted to these prostate conditions.

This chapter will provide you with what is essential to know in terms of prostate-healthy and prostate-unhealthy foods.

MEDITERRANEAN DIET TO THE RESCUE

I am a big proponent of the Mediterranean diet. It has been shown in several studies to be protective against prostate cancer. Furthermore, the high amounts of plant foods, herbs, and spices serve to keep the prostate healthy. However, I recommend modifying the traditional guidelines in order to reduce dairy as well as grain products. Most American grain products, such as breads and pastas, are so refined and unhealthy that I recommend eliminating them if possible. Even "healthier" whole grains, however, should be eaten in moderation.

As explained in Chapter 5, the Mediterranean diet consists of plenty of plant foods (fruits, vegetables, legumes, nuts, breads, and unrefined cereals); lots of olive oil; moderately high intake of fish; moderate consumption of alcohol; and low consumption of poultry, red meat, and eggs.[2]

This diet is also rich in omega-3 fatty acids, as found in cold-water fish. These healthy omega-3s reduce inflammatory compounds that are related to BPH.[3] Research has shown that blood levels of omega-3 fatty acids were significantly decreased in men with BPH.[4]

Harvard Medical School provides great tips for incorporating the Mediterranean diet into your meals:[5]

- Eat more nuts and olives.

- Begin or end each meal with a salad.

- Add a variety of different vegetables to the menu.

- Eat at least three servings a week of legumes (e.g., lentils, chickpeas, beans, peas).

- Reach for wine if you choose to drink alcoholic beverages (but limit yourself to no more than two five-ounce glasses a day).

HEALTHY FATS

While the main fat used in the Mediterranean diet is olive oil, it is not the only one I believe can be part of a healthy diet. In general, I recommend the following:

Fats to include: extra-virgin olive oil, avocado oil, coconut oil, macadamia nut oil

Fats to avoid: butter

REDUCE YOUR DAIRY CONSUMPTION

I recommend a diet that is restricted in cow's milk products because they have potential inflammatory effects. Furthermore, most of the world's population is actually lactose intolerant. Some people have found, however, that they are able to tolerate small amounts of dairy products from sheep and goats rather than cows.

Healthier alternatives include unsweetened plant-based "milk" from the following:

- oat
- cashew
- almond
- coconut
- hazelnut
- hemp

LIMIT YOUR SUGAR INTAKE— INCLUDING THE ONES FROM GRAINS!

It's best to follow a diet low in simple sugars to reduce inflammation and avoid immune suppression. Cut out sugary beverages. Eat fewer high-fat, high-sugar desserts.

The World Health Organization recommends consuming less than 5 percent of one's calories from added sugar, natural sugars in honey, as well as sugar from sweetened beverages and fruit juice. This means that added sugar should be less than 25 grams per day—but most Americans consume 82 grams daily.[6]

Obvious simple sugars found in pastries, candies, cookies, and soda should be avoided. However, research has shown that most of the grains that Americans consume are high glycemic. In other words, they spike blood sugar and insulin levels. This contributes greatly to insulin resistance, prediabetes, and diabetes. Also, insulin resistance increases estrogen levels, an enemy of good prostate health and men's health in general.[7] (It's important to note here that while fruit is high in sugar, studies have found that fruit consumed in its whole, natural form is not related to insulin resistance.)

In general, restrict "white" processed grain products. Seek out products that are made with whole grains or alternatives that make them high in fiber and protein such as quinoa pasta and brown rice pasta. High-fiber breads like "Paleo bread" and Ezekiel brand bread are also good choices.

INCREASE YOUR CONSUMPTION OF POLYPHENOLS WITH POWER PLANTS

Plant foods form the backbone of a prostate-friendly diet thanks to their wealth of phytonutrients such as polyphenols, a group of antioxidants found in plants that have anti-inflammatory effects. According to a 2017 article in *Frontiers in Pharmacology*, the prostate is one of the bodily tissues where polyphenols make a real impact.[8]

Many fruits and vegetables contain a variety of polyphenols. Examples of foods rich in polyphenols include red wine, red grape juice, legumes, turmeric, and green tea. There is research on prostate health and polyphenols such as flaxseed lignans, lycopene from tomatoes, and soybean isoflavones. Interestingly, dietary polyphenols have 5-alpha-reductase-inhibitory properties.[9] Inhibiting 5-alpha-reductase is a key mechanism for treating BPH.

Smoothies and juices are a great way to increase your consumption of fruits' and vegetables' protective polyphenols. Make them with fresh, organic, seasonal produce, such as apples in the fall and strawberries in the spring and summer. Include peels when edible, as with apples and carrots.

Conventional fruit juices are usually highly processed and loaded with sugar, and therefore should be avoided. However, when making juices at home, you may end up with a sugary beverage as well if you're not careful. Include vegetables along with your fruit to balance the sweetness: try mostly spinach, kale, or another leafy green with smaller amounts of a sweet fruit like apple or mango for antioxidants and flavor. Many juicers strip fruits of their fiber; I recommend using a high-speed blender instead of a juicer so you include the fiber along with the flesh.

BOOST YOUR FIBER INTAKE

Plant foods, of course, are your source of fiber, which promotes hormone balance and digestive health and has anticancer properties. If you struggle with consuming five to nine servings of fruits and vegetables daily, then consider making a vegetable/fruit smoothie blend.

Also, consider regular use of organic ground flaxseed at a dose of one to two tablespoons daily added to shakes, salads, cereals, or baked goods. Make sure to drink 8 to 10 ounces of water with this high-fiber superfood for easier consumption. Research shows that supplementing the diet with ground flaxseed is safe and may be protective against prostate cancer.[10]

GET RED IN YOUR DIET

Lycopene, a well-known prostate superfood, is an antioxidant that is found in abundance in red fruits and vegetables. According to an article published in *Medicine*, higher circulating levels of lycopene significantly reduce the risk of prostate cancer.

Protect your prostate by increasing your consumption of tomatoes (which are plentiful in the Mediterranean diet), watermelon, and pink grapefruits. To ensure that lycopene is most available to the body, be sure to eat plenty of cooked rather than raw tomatoes, as heating releases lycopene to be used by the body.

DRINK GREEN TEA

Green tea, made from the fresh leaves of *Camellia sinensis*, contains polyphenols that are composed of catechins. Several studies have shown that the major polyphenol in green tea exhibits anticancer activity. (See Chapter 5 for more detail.) I recommend that you drink as many cups of organic green tea as is tolerable or as recommended by your integrative doctor.

CAREFUL WITH THE GRILLED MEAT

The question of meat consumption and disease always brings up a lively debate. In terms of prostate health, it makes sense to limit meat products and preferably stick to grass-fed or organic.

Most importantly, limit the intake of well-done meats that are grilled due to the carcinogens (heterocyclic amines and polycyclic aromatic hydrocarbons) that are created when meats are cooked at high temperatures. Studies are not consistent on this matter, but some studies have indicated an association between cancer risk and well-cooked meat.[11]

If you do grill or fry meat, then consider the following recommendations from the Institute for Functional Medicine:[12]

- Use lean meat such as grass-fed steak, chicken (remove the skin), or fish instead of fatty burgers.

- Avoid charring and trim charred portions of meat. Rotate the meat frequently so the center cooks without overheating the surface.

- Use antioxidant-rich, acidic marinades, which may reduce the number of carcinogenic heterocyclic amines that are produced. (Some herbs that have been found to be protective include garlic, ginger, thyme, and rosemary.)

EAT HEALTHFULLY

Obesity, especially central obesity with increased waist circumference, is a known risk factor for BPH and prostate cancer. There are several mechanisms by which being overweight increases your risk of these common prostate diseases, such as increased intra-abdominal pressure, altered hormone balance, imbalanced nervous system activity, increased inflammation, and damaging oxidative stress.[13]

Make sure you are not only eating healthier but consuming an appropriate amount for your size and activity level as well. If your calorie intake is less than what you are expending activity-wise, then your weight should be reducing. Check in with your care providers as to a nutrition and exercise plan that suits your health needs. Other factors such as hormone balance can play a role in metabolism as well, so your doctors may want to run a few tests to check your thyroid, among other factors.

GO ORGANIC

Seek out the best-quality food available (farmer's markets for locally grown, seasonal foods). Consider organic foods whenever possible. According to a 2019 study from the Environmental Working Group and the Department of Agriculture,[14] almost 70 percent of produce sold in the United States is tainted with pesticide residues. These residues can include synthetic xenoestrogens,[15] which are endocrine disruptors and can cause adverse effects by mimicking estrogen in the body.[16] According to a 2008 article in *Endocrine-Related Cancer,* "There is increasing evidence . . . that specific endocrine-disrupting compounds may influence the development or progression of prostate cancer. . . . In humans, epidemiologic evidence links specific pesticides, PCBs and inorganic arsenic exposures to elevated prostate cancer risk."[17]

The Environmental Working Group releases a "Dirty Dozen" each year, describing the fruits and vegetables with the most pesticides. The list for 2020 includes strawberries, spinach, kale, nectarines, apples, grapes, peaches, cherries, pears, tomatoes, celery, and potatoes.[18] If you are not able to purchase only organic produce, this list is a good place to focus on.

Similarly, when buying canned products (such as beans or tomato sauce), look for items in BPA-free packaging. This is important because bisphenol A is a synthetic xenoestrogen that can negatively influence prostate cancer cells.[19]

CONSIDER FASTING

A growing body of research shows the advantages of intermittent fasting. The term refers to eating cycle patterns in which a person does not consume any food for a period. There are many techniques for intermittent fasting, but most guidelines include consuming water only for a period of 10 to 16 hours a day, one to seven days a week. (Don't be daunted—this time period includes when you sleep, so successful intermittent fasting can be as simple as delaying your breakfast.)

Another popular method is choosing two days a week to consume only one moderate-sized meal for the day. The rest of the week, you eat as normal.

Timing is vital with intermittent fasting. Research stresses the importance of not eating late in the evening. Intermittent fasting can help weight loss and insulin sensitivity and may have anticancer properties.[20]

There are many different recommendations around intermittent fasting. If you are interested in learning more, I include recommendations for further research in my online resources guide at www.markstengler.com.

Main Takeaways from This Chapter

- Follow a Mediterranean diet, with limited amounts of grains and dairy.

- Reduce your animal protein intake.

- Eat five to nine servings of vegetables a day (in a smoothie, if necessary).

- Consume one to two tablespoons flaxseed daily (along with 8 to 10 ounces of water).

- Eat lycopene-rich foods, such as tomatoes, watermelon, and pink grapefruits. Cooked tomatoes are higher in lycopene than raw.

- Drink as much green tea a day as tolerated, or as recommended by your integrative doctor.

- Limit the amount of foods you eat that are grilled or cooked at a high heat.

- Watch your caloric intake to maintain a healthy weight and body fat ratio.

- Eat organic foods whenever possible.

- Make sure your canned products are in BPA-free packaging.

- Consider intermittent fasting.

CHAPTER 9

KEY FACTORS FOR MEN'S HEALTH

You have read a lot of updated scientific information about how to improve your prostate health in this book, *Healing the Prostate*. There are many specific things you can do through diet and lifestyle changes, prostate-specific nutraceuticals, and hormone balancing, as well as conventional therapies, to be proactive in achieving prostate wellness.

It is important to keep in mind that the prostate gland is one of many parts of an entire body system. One area where holistic and integrative medicine shines is recognizing the fact that each small system of the body is affected by other parts of the body's systems. For example, you learned how hormone imbalance occurs through problems with diet, environmental toxins, the functioning of your detoxification organs (liver and kidneys), and the chemical communication system of glands in your body. When hormone imbalance occurs, it causes imbalanced signaling to the receptors of the prostate gland, which can lead to growth and problems such as BPH or prostate cancer. So to treat just the prostate gland by itself (the conventional approach) is an incomplete and reductionist way of preventing and treating prostate problems.

In this chapter, I will review additional holistic support you can use to counter the effects of stress. This is important in maintaining a healthy inflammatory state, hormone balance, immune system, and prostate. I will also review important information on gut health, environmental toxins, and detoxification that is essential for a healthy body, hormonal system, and prostate. These recommendations are of course to be used in conjunction with the healthy diet, exercise, and hormone-balancing protocols already reviewed in detail in this book.

THE TELOMERE FACTOR

Telomeres are protective, repeated units of nucleotides (letters of coding) at the tips of chromosomes (strands of DNA that encode your genetic information). The telomeres prevent the long strands of genetic material from wearing down or being destroyed, allowing your cells to divide properly. An enzyme known as telomerase has several functions, one of which is to maintain telomere length and gene stability. The length of telomeres and telomerase activity are important factors for susceptibility to diseases such as cancer and possibly aging.

A review in *Psychoneuroendocrinology* found that 13 out of 14 studies on lifestyle factors demonstrated that exercise, nutrient supplementation (omega-3, lycopene, lutein, zeaxanthin, selenium, vitamin D, vitamin E), mindfulness meditation, qigong practice or yoga meditation resulted in increased telomerase activity. The same researchers also found that there was decreased telomerase activity in individuals under chronic stress.[1] A separate study found that adults who frequently attend church services, pray with regularity, and consider themselves to be religious tend to have longer telomeres than those who attend and pray less frequently and do not consider themselves to be religious.[2]

More specifically, a study was done on integrative lifestyle intervention and telomerase activity in 30 men with low-risk prostate cancer. The study involved a three-month intervention of a low-fat, plant-based diet; moderate aerobic exercise (walking 30 minutes a day, six days a week); yoga-based stretching, meditation, imagery, and progressive relaxation (60 minutes per day for six days a week); and a one-hour group support session once a week. Telomerase activity was found to increase significantly for the participants.[3]

So you can see that what people do with their diet, lifestyle, and stress-reduction techniques impacts their cells even at the DNA level. Do not underestimate the controllable factors that you have available to impact your body and overall health.

STRESS

As you know, stress seems to play a role in most health problems. With short-term stress, our adrenal glands (located on top of our kidneys) respond to a messaging system from the brain and release epinephrine (adrenaline) and norepinephrine (noradrenaline), which act as both hormones and neurotransmitters (molecules having both actions are known as neurohormones). The short-term response of epinephrine and norepinephrine through nervous system messaging increases heart rate and blood pressure, stimulates the liver to break down glycogen to glucose and releases it into the blood for energy supply, dilates bronchioles, reduces digestion and urination, and increases metabolic rate.

In response to long-term stress, the brain sends messaging to the adrenal glands to release hormones such as dehydroepiandrosterone (DHEA) and cortisol. Both DHEA and cortisol reduce inflammation and immune activity. However, prolonged elevation of cortisol levels is detrimental to your health and increases the risk of anxiety, depression, digestive problems, headaches, heart disease, sleep problems, weight gain, memory and concentration impairment, and even cancer.[4]

In terms of the prostate and stress, a study examining the relationship between psychological stress and BPH was conducted on a group of 83 men with BPH. The researchers concluded based on the results of the study that higher physiological stress responses in laboratory testing in men with BPH are associated with more severe BPH disease.[5]

Researchers from Sweden surveyed 4,105 men being treated for localized prostate cancer and found those with the highest levels of perceived stress had a 66 percent higher risk of mortality compared to men with low stress levels.[6]

The American Society of Clinical Oncology gives the following tips, which can apply to men with any type of health condition, for reducing and managing stress:[7]

- Avoid scheduling conflicts
- Be aware of your limits
- Ask for help
- Prioritize your tasks
- Break down tasks into smaller steps

- Concentrate your efforts on things you can control

- Get help with financial problems

- Exercise regularly

- Spend time outside

- Schedule social activities

- Eat well

- Get plenty of sleep

- Join a support group

- Schedule daily relaxing time

- Do things you enjoy

- Write in a journal

- Learn a new hobby

Herbal Adaptogens for Stress

Specific herbal extracts can be used to support the body in balancing stress hormones and becoming more resilient to the effects of stress. Herbal adaptogens are excellent for this purpose. The European Medicines Agency (EMA) has defined herbal adaptogens as those substances that "have the capacity to normalize body functions and strengthen systems compromised by stress. They are reported to have a protective effect on health against a wide variety of environmental assaults and emotional conditions."[8]

Two of the top herbal adaptogens that men have access to are ashwagandha and *Rhodiola rosea*.

- *Ashwagandha* has a long history of use in Ayurvedic medicine. It has had several human studies published concerning its beneficial effects as an adaptogen.

  Ashwagandha extract was shown in people with a history of chronic stress to improve an individual's stress resistance and quality-of-life scores based on a variety of questionnaires. The participants' perceived stress was reduced by 44 percent. In addition, after 60 days, serum cortisol levels were reduced by 27.9 percent from baseline compared to 7.9 percent among those in the placebo group.[9] Also, a double-blind, placebo-controlled trial found that 125 to 250 mg of ashwagandha extract taken twice daily resulted in a 79 percent reduction in fatigue. There were also reductions in stress, anxiety, irritability, inability to concentrate, and forgetfulness. These factors did not improve in the placebo group. Furthermore, serum cortisol levels decreased by 24.2 percent, and DHEA levels increased by 32.2 percent, for those taking ashwagandha extract.[10] In addition, in a study of 20 healthy males, ashwagandha extract supplementation of 500 mg twice daily resulted in significant improvement in the subjects' reaction time, attention span, response speed, visual-motor coordination, alertness levels, and integrative and executive functions.[11]

  Recommendation: 250 to 500 mg daily of a standardized extract

  Safety: Ashwagandha is well tolerated.

- *Rhodiola rosea* is a medicinal plant that has
  had several studies published on its chemistry
  and clinical use. It has a long history of
  use in Siberian and Russian medicine as an
  adaptogen. It also functions as an effective
  antioxidant that protects the brain and
  nervous system from free radical damage.
  Rhodiola has been shown to increase physical
  work capacity and shorten recovery time
  between bouts of high-intensity exercise.[12]
  A review in the journal *Current
  Pharmacology Reports* states that recent
  research demonstrates that *Rhodiola
  rosea* has "anti-aging, anti-inflammation,
  immunostimulating, DNA repair and anti-
  cancer effects in different model systems."[13]
  Moreover, the authors of a paper from the
  *International Journal of Psychiatry in Clinical
  Practice* found that *Rhodiola rosea* extract
  has the beneficial actions of "providing
  both physical and psychological symptom
  relief, normalising stress hormone levels
  and increasing energy."[14] Also, rhodiola
  has beneficial effects on neurotransmitter
  production in the brain and balancing effects
  on the hypothalamic-pituitary-adrenal axis.[15]
  Recommendation: 200 to 300 mg
  of a standardized product containing 3
  percent rosavins
  Safety: Side effects with rhodiola
  are uncommon.

The following nutrients support healthy adrenal gland function. They can be used in addition to a high-quality multivitamin and mineral formula:[16]

- vitamin C (1000 to 2000 mg)

- pantothenic acid (also known as vitamin B5) (100 to 250 mg)

- magnesium (250 to 500 mg)

GUT HEALTH

Central to the idea of whole-body health is healthy digestion and detoxification. A healthy digestive and detoxification system works to control inflammation in the body. Most of your body's immune system and neurotransmitter production originate in the gut tissues.

Assuming that your diet is healthy, the next critical step is good digestion, which involves the breakdown and absorption of food, and then proper elimination of waste materials.

Good digestive health begins with eating in an atmosphere conducive to a calm nervous system. This means eating in a relaxed atmosphere where you are not rushed. Chew your food thoroughly before swallowing.

If you have digestive problems such as IBS, IBD, or acid reflux, then it is important you work with an integrative doctor to heal your digestive system. A healthy digestive system means a healthy body. Digestive enzymes, probiotics, and digestion-specific herbals can do wonders for improving digestive function. They also help with hormone balance and reducing inflammation. If you are one of the millions of Americans taking proton pump inhibitors (PPIs) for acid reflux, then you should know you are at risk for nutritional deficiencies. Your stomach acid not only helps to break down protein and liquefy other foodstuffs but is of critical importance for the absorption of nutrients, including magnesium, B12, calcium, iron, and vitamin C.[17] While PPIs can help your symptoms, they are not treating the root cause of your acid reflux. Furthermore, modern research has shown that long-term use of PPIs is not safe. [18]

DETOXIFICATION

The importance of detoxification cannot be overstated. We live in a world in which many tens of thousands of human-made chemicals are present in the environment. The President's Cancer Panel states, "With nearly 80,000 chemicals on the market in the United States, many of which are used by millions of Americans in their daily lives and are un- or understudied and largely unregulated, exposure to potential environmental carcinogens is widespread."[19]

I discussed in Chapter 6 the science on how endocrine-disrupting chemicals (EDCs) from the environment affect the function of the testes. The prostate and other organs of the body are affected by endocrine-disrupting chemicals as well. Examples of EDCs include pesticides, insecticides, plasticizers such as BPA and BPB, and phthalates. A study of nearly 2,000 men who developed prostate cancer found a significant association between cancer and prolonged exposure to workplace chemicals (used in the manufacturing of polymers, rubber products, or shoes, as well as painting, leather tanning, and printing) that included benzene, toluene, xylene, and styrene.[20]

One of the best things you can do is to avoid exposure to substances that are known toxins when you can help it. This is done by eating organic foods as much as possible, drinking filtered water, using nontoxic household cleaners, and reducing exposure to electromagnetic radiation as much as possible (e.g., direct cell phone use, etc.).

The use of holistic techniques to support detoxification is essential for good health. In addition to a healthy diet and exercise, the use of nutraceuticals that support detoxification pathways is essential.

Also, sauna therapy on a regular basis aids the body in eliminating toxins through sweating. One sauna session a week can make a difference over several months in terms of detoxification.

Supplements for Detoxification

Glutathione is one of the body's most important antioxidants that supports cellular detoxification and has functions for the liver and kidney cells. Glutathione is found in foods such as apples, avocado, watermelon, asparagus, broccoli, raw carrots, spinach, and raw tomatoes. You need about 300 mg daily, but most Americans consume about half that amount. Glutathione can also be used in supplement form, or the body's levels can be increased from supplements of vitamin C (1000 mg/daily), milk thistle (500 mg/daily), and N-acetylcysteine (500 mg/daily). Supplemental dosages of studied forms of glutathione range from 250 to 1000 mg daily.

Herbs that support liver and kidney detoxification are very helpful and easily found in liver formulas. The common ones used include milk thistle, dandelion root, turmeric, and artichoke. Use as directed on the label. These types of formulas can be used under your integrative doctor's supervision.

Sweating Out Toxins

Additionally, therapies that promote sweating are helpful to promote regular detoxification. The use of a variety of saunas can be effective in supporting detoxification.

◆ ◆ ◆

In summary, by incorporating the protocols I recommend in reducing the effects of stress and supporting good digestion and detoxification, you will go a long way toward not just feeling better but also creating an environment that promotes hormone balance and good prostate health.

These protocols will not only improve prostate and hormonal health, but they often invigorate the whole body as evidenced by improved energy, clarity of mind, mood, and immunity. Use these approaches to your advantage and take action. Most men will notice a dramatic improvement in their health!

APPENDIX
Two-Week Meal Plan and Recipes

In general, I recommend a modified Mediterranean diet full of organic plant foods (especially fruits and vegetables), free of dairy, and low in animal products. That is the basis of the following two-week meal plan.

This plan is meant to give you an idea of the wide variety of foods you can have on a modified Mediterranean diet. Following the meal plan, I've also included recipes for some of the more complex dishes. If you need more recipes and meal-planning ideas, please see my website www.markstengler.com.

Day 1
Breakfast: Oatmeal prepared with nondairy milk such as cashew or almond, toasted nuts, and fresh and dried fruit
Lunch: Roasted beet salad with chickpeas, greens, and toasted walnuts
Dinner: Cauliflower steaks with tahini sauce, toasted walnuts, and pomegranate seeds, served with Moroccan-spiced roasted carrots (carrot recipe in this chapter)
Snack: Smoothie with frozen bananas, peanut butter, and almond milk

Day 2

Breakfast: Brown rice porridge with chia seeds, topped with fresh citrus

Lunch: Almond butter and fresh blueberry sandwich on whole-grain bread

Dinner: Chicken soup with whole-wheat pasta or zucchini noodles

Snack: Nondairy yogurt topped with banana slices

Day 3

Breakfast: Cranberry-ginger juice and tofu scramble with *pico de gallo* (tomato-onion salsa)

Lunch: Grilled chicken salad with tomatoes, cucumber, and balsamic vinaigrette

Dinner: Roasted sweet potato half topped with black beans (or chicken) and roasted vegetables

Snack: Smoothie with frozen berries, almond butter, and nondairy milk

Day 4

Breakfast: Whole-wheat (or gluten-free) toast with mashed avocado and white beans

Lunch: Black bean soup with cumin and oregano (recipe in this chapter)

Dinner: Turkey-apple burgers with mustard, with baked sweet potato fries

Snack: Tangerine and a handful of toasted nuts

Day 5

Breakfast: Egg-white omelet with broccoli, tomatoes, and onions, served with tomato sauce

Lunch: Fried cauliflower "rice" with tofu or tempeh, carrots, bell peppers, onions, garlic, and ginger

Dinner: Chicken fajitas with sautéed bell peppers and onions

Snack: Carrot sticks with carrot-miso dressing (recipe in this chapter)

Day 6
Breakfast: Whole-grain banana-blueberry pancakes (recipe in this chapter)
Lunch: Black beans and brown rice with pico de gallo and guacamole
Dinner: Curried tofu and peas in tomato sauce
Snack: Mango and tahini smoothie (recipe in this chapter)

Day 7
Breakfast: Tempeh stir-fry with bell peppers, onion, ginger, and garlic
Lunch: Creamy tuna and chickpea spread (recipe in this chapter) with fresh vegetables and whole-wheat toast
Dinner: Sweet potato and pinto bean chili with guacamole
Snack: Apple slices with almond butter

Day 8
Breakfast: Grape-lime juice, smoked salmon, and avocado toast
Lunch: Tabbouleh salad with chickpeas
Dinner: Turkey-corn-tomato sauté (recipe in this chapter)
Snack: Kale chips (recipe in this chapter)

Day 9
Breakfast: Grapefruit-turmeric juice and whole-wheat toast with almond butter
Lunch: Edamame, bell pepper, cucumber, cashew salad with carrot-ginger dressing
Dinner: Black bean chili served with quinoa
Snack: Roasted spiced chickpeas

Day 10
Breakfast: Sweet potato "toast" drizzled with tahini and topped with fresh berries
Lunch: Chickpea and brown rice salad with raisins, green onion, and bell peppers
Dinner: Veggie burgers with pinto beans, carrots, and whole-wheat bread crumbs
Snack: Edamame

Day 11

Breakfast: Apple-ginger juice and toasted nuts with nondairy yogurt

Lunch: Roast salmon and vegetables served with farro

Dinner: Stuffed baked squash with black beans and vegetables

Snack: Celery sticks with peanut butter and raisins

Day 12

Breakfast: Chickpeas simmered in tomato sauce, topped with nondairy yogurt

Lunch: Open-faced tempeh and vegetable sandwich on whole-wheat bread

Dinner: Lettuce wraps with sautéed ground chicken flavored with soy sauce, garlic, and ginger

Snack: Avocado and citrus salad

Day 13

Breakfast: Open-faced sandwich with one fried egg, black beans, avocado, and fresh tomato

Lunch: Lentil soup with nondairy yogurt

Dinner: Salmon cakes with yogurt-dill sauce (recipe in this chapter)

Snack: Frozen grapes and toasted walnuts

Day 14

Breakfast: Oatmeal topped with chunky spiced pear sauce (recipe for sauce in this chapter) and toasted nuts

Lunch: Whole-wheat (or gluten-free) wrap with hummus, bean sprouts, cucumber, and tomato

Dinner: Roasted tofu, baby tomatoes, and eggplant drizzled with balsamic vinegar

Snack: Baked spiced apple topped with nondairy yogurt and toasted nuts

RECIPES

Prostate Super Juice

Makes 1½ cups (serves 1)

Green in hue, this slightly vegetal, slightly sweet juice includes fruits and vegetables that protect the prostate and taste delicious. Be sure to use canned or cooked tomatoes, since they feature lycopene in the form most bioavailable to the body.

½ cup fresh kale leaves
½ cup fresh spinach leaves
½ cup thinly sliced carrot
¼ cup unsweetened pomegranate juice
¼ cup diced tomatoes with juice
⅛ teaspoon salt

Add all of the ingredients plus ½ cup water to a high-speed blender. Puree until smooth, 1 to 2 minutes.

◆ ◆ ◆

Anti-Inflammatory Carrot-Apple Juice

Makes 1 cup (serves 1)

This sweet, orange-hued juice features ingredients that help combat prostate inflammation.

1 cup diced sweet apple, such as Pink Lady (unpeeled)
½ cup thinly sliced carrot
¼ cup fresh orange juice
1 coin peeled fresh ginger root (about ¼ teaspoon)
¼ teaspoon salt
⅛ teaspoon ground turmeric

Add all of the ingredients plus ¼ cup water to a high-speed blender. Puree until smooth, 1 to 2 minutes.

Mango and Tahini Smoothie

Makes 2 cups (serves 1 to 2)

Mango, tahini, and almond milk supply antioxidants in this sweet, creamy snack or treat. Be sure to use extra-ripe fresh mangoes, as frozen versions won't be sufficiently sweet. The fresh mangoes should be so ripe as to give a lot when squeezed.

1 large very ripe mango, pitted, peeled, and chopped (about 1½ cups flesh)
1 cup plain, unsweetened plant milk, such as almond milk
3 ice cubes
2 tablespoons tahini
¼ teaspoon vanilla extract
⅛ teaspoon salt

Add all of these ingredients to a blender, and puree until smooth.

◆ ◆ ◆

Whole-Grain Banana-Blueberry Pancakes

Makes 20 to 24 pancakes (serves about 6)

This recipe is free of sweeteners. For the ultimate in flavor, opt for extra-ripe bananas. They should be brown and give a lot when squeezed. I tend to keep ripe bananas in my refrigerator for recipes like this one. If you can't find ground flaxseed meal, purchase whole flaxseeds and grind in a spice grinder. White whole-wheat flour features a milder, lighter-hued variety of wheat; however, if you can't find it, just go with traditional whole-wheat flour. Gluten-free flours are available for those who are gluten-free.

2 cups whole-wheat or white whole-wheat flour
   (or gluten-free flour)
½ cup ground flaxseed meal
2 teaspoons baking powder
1 teaspoon ground cinnamon
1 teaspoon sea or kosher salt
4 medium extra-ripe bananas, peeled
1½ cups plain or vanilla unsweetened plant milk,
   such as cashew milk
4 large organic eggs
¼ cup extra-virgin olive oil, plus about another
   ¼ cup for cooking
2 teaspoons vanilla extract
2 cups blueberries, rinsed and patted dry

Combine the first five ingredients in a medium bowl. Whisk well.

In a large bowl, mash the bananas well with a potato masher. Add the plant milk, eggs, oil, and vanilla, and stir well. Pour in the dry mixture, and stir well with a wooden spoon.

Brush a nonstick griddle pan with a thin coating of olive oil, and heat over medium heat. When hot, add the batter in ¼-cup dollops, spacing the pancakes apart. Sprinkle each pancake with 4 or 5 blueberries. Cook until the undersides of the pancakes are golden brown and cooked through, 3 to 4 minutes.

Flip and cook the other sides until golden brown and cooked through, about another 3 minutes. Repeat with the remaining batter and blueberries.

❖ ❖ ❖

Black Bean Soup with Cumin and Oregano

Makes 6 cups (serves 3)

Full of antioxidant-rich black beans, vegetables, and citrus, this creamy vegan soup is satisfying and low in fat. Feel free to top with a dollop of plain, unsweetened plant-based yogurt, such as cashew yogurt.

- 1 tablespoon extra-virgin olive oil
- 1 medium red onion, chopped (about 2 cups)
- 1 medium orange or yellow bell pepper, chopped (about 1 cup)
- 4 teaspoons sliced garlic (about 5 cloves)
- 1 teaspoon cumin
- 1 teaspoon oregano
- One 29-ounce BPA-free can black beans, rinsed and drained
- 3 cups low-sodium vegetable broth or stock
- ½ cup fresh orange juice
- 1 teaspoon salt

Heat the oil in a medium pot over medium-high heat. Once hot, add the onion, bell pepper, garlic, cumin, and oregano, and sauté until the onion is soft, about 8 minutes (do not let the vegetables brown). Stir in the beans, broth, juice, and salt, and bring to a boil over high heat.

Once boiling, cover the pot and reduce the heat to medium-low. Simmer for 20 minutes. Then, using an immersion blender, carefully puree in the pot until smooth. Alternatively, you may puree in batches in a blender.

◆ ◆ ◆

Garlic Roasted Tofu
with Cabbage and Onion

Makes 6 tofu rectangles (serves 2)

Thanks to soybeans, cabbage, onions, and tomato sauce, this entrée delivers a lot of protective polyphenols. The tofu is so versatile in terms of flavor, it can pair with virtually any condiment. That said, I recommend serving it with warmed-up store-bought marinara sauce (choose a brand without sugar) for the lycopene.

Coconut or olive oil cooking spray
1 pound organic extra-firm high-protein tofu,
  cut into 6 rectangles (each about ½ inch thick)
½ teaspoon garlic powder
1 teaspoon salt, divided
¼ teaspoon ground black pepper
5 cups thinly chopped cabbage (about ½ medium
  head of cabbage)
1 cup chopped red onion (about ½ medium onion)
2 tablespoons extra-virgin olive oil
For serving: about ⅓ cup marinara sauce, warmed-up

Preheat oven to 425°F and line a large baking sheet with foil. Spray the foil with cooking spray. Place the tofu rectangles on one half of the baking sheet. Sprinkle both sides of the tofu evenly with the garlic powder, ½ teaspoon of the salt, and the pepper. Spray the tofu with the cooking spray, and roast in the oven for 10 minutes.

Meanwhile, in a large bowl, toss the cabbage and onion with the remaining ½ teaspoon salt and the olive oil. When the tofu comes out of the oven, carefully spread the vegetable mixture in one layer onto the other side of the baking sheet. Continue roasting until the vegetables are tender, with some pieces golden brown, and the tofu is slightly golden brown—about 20 minutes. Serve with warm marinara sauce.

◆ ◆ ◆

Turkey-Corn-Tomato Sauté

Makes 10 cups (serves about 5)

Similar to a sloppy joe mixture (but without the added sugar), this quick-to-prepare entrée is loaded with antioxidant-rich tomatoes and corn. Lean turkey is a healthful way to glean protein—without the saturated fat found in so many meats. Serve this dish with cooked whole grains such as brown rice or even on a slice of whole-grain toast. I like to prepare the entire batch, which is ideal for families or casual gatherings.

    2 tablespoons avocado oil, divided
    2 pounds 99% lean ground turkey or chicken
    2½ teaspoons cumin, divided
    2½ teaspoons garlic powder, divided
    1½ teaspoons salt, divided
    2 cups small-diced red and orange bell peppers
        (about 2 peppers)
    1¼ cups small-diced red onion (about 1 small onion)
    4 teaspoons thinly sliced garlic
    One 28-ounce BPA-free can whole peeled plum tomatoes
    One 15-ounce BPA-free can cooked corn kernels

Heat half of the oil in a 10- to 12-inch nonstick sauté pan with a minimum of 2-inch-high sides over medium-high heat. When the oil is hot, add the turkey in one layer, 2 teaspoons each of the cumin and garlic powder, and 1 teaspoon of the salt. Sauté, breaking the meat up often with a wooden spoon, until it becomes opaque, about 8 minutes. Set the cooked turkey aside.

Add the remaining oil and the bell pepper, onion, garlic, and remaining ½ teaspoon each of salt, garlic powder, and cumin to the pan. Sauté until the pepper is soft, about 12 minutes.

Add the tomatoes and crush a bit with a potato masher. Stir in the corn. Increase the heat to high and cook, stirring, for about 3 minutes.

Salmon Cakes with Yogurt-Dill Sauce

Makes 10 cakes and a scant 1 cup sauce (serves about 5)

Wild salmon provides healthy omega-3 fats and protein. For an added boost of polyphenols, serve over a large salad with cucumber, arugula, and tomato. Unlike typical salmon cake recipes, this version is extremely low in saturated fat (thanks to the absence of mayonnaise and the use of extra-virgin olive oil). I like to prepare the full recipe, then freeze the extra salmon cakes and defrost them before using them.

For the cakes
2 large eggs
2 14.75-ounce BPA-free cans wild salmon
1 cup minced red onion
1 cup whole-wheat bread crumbs
3 tablespoons minced fresh dill
3 tablespoons extra-virgin olive oil, plus about another 3
    tablespoons for cooking
1 tablespoon dijon mustard
1 teaspoon salt

For the sauce
½ cup plain, unsweetened plant-based yogurt, such as cashew
¼ cup grated cucumber flesh
2 tablespoons minced red onion
1 tablespoon capers, rinsed
1 tablespoon white balsamic vinegar
¼ teaspoon salt

To make the cakes: In a medium-large bowl, whisk the eggs. Add the salmon, onion, bread crumbs, dill, 3 tablespoons of the oil, mustard, and salt. Use your hands to knead together. With a ½-cup measure, form 10 cakes.

Heat 1 tablespoon of olive oil in a medium nonstick pan over medium-high heat. Once hot, add 4 of the cakes and cook until golden brown on the undersides, about 3 minutes. Flip and cook until other sides are golden brown, about another 3 minutes. Set aside. Repeat with the remaining cakes in two more batches, greasing the pan with about 1 tablespoon more oil before each batch.

To make the sauce: In a small-medium bowl, stir together all of the sauce ingredients. Serve with the salmon cakes.

◆ ◆ ◆

Moroccan-Spiced Roasted Carrots

Makes about 5 cups (serves 4)

Carrots are one of the plant foods most associated with benefits for the prostate (plus, they taste delicious). This recipe jazzes them up with Middle Eastern spices, raisins, and a touch of honey. For ease, purchase bags of "baby" carrots, which are actually full-size carrots that have been cut into smaller pieces. Make sure the honey is runny, rather than crystallized.

> Olive or coconut oil cooking spray
> 5 cups "baby" carrots
> ¼ cup fresh orange juice
> 1 tablespoon extra-virgin olive oil
> 1 teaspoon salt
> 1 teaspoon garlic powder
> ½ teaspoon cinnamon
> ½ teaspoon cumin
> ¼ teaspoon cayenne
> ¼ cup raisins
> 1 teaspoon honey

Preheat oven to 400°F and line a large baking sheet with foil. Spray the foil with the cooking spray. In a large bowl, toss the carrots with the juice, oil, salt, garlic powder, cinnamon, cumin, and cayenne. Pour onto the baking sheet in one layer. Roast until tender, about 40 minutes.

Meanwhile, 10 minutes before the carrots are done, soak the raisins in very hot water. Then drain.

Pour the cooked carrots into a medium bowl, along with the drained raisins and honey. Toss with tongs.

◆ ◆ ◆

Kale Chips

Makes 4 cups (serves 2)

This addictive snack—starring a cruciferous vegetable—is at its most crunchy and appealing when served warm from the oven. If you chill or eat these later on, they won't be as crispy. For an extra flavor boost, feel free to sprinkle with spices such as crushed red pepper flakes, sesame seeds, or garlic powder.

6 cups chopped kale leaves, stems removed (about 1 bunch)
2 tablespoons extra-virgin olive oil
¼ teaspoon salt

Preheat oven to 350°F and line a large baking sheet with parchment paper or aluminum foil (if the latter, grease the foil with olive oil cooking spray).

In a large bowl, use your hands to toss the kale with the oil and salt. Spread in one layer onto a baking sheet.

Bake until crisp, about 30 minutes. Serve immediately.

◆ ◆ ◆

Creamy Tuna and Chickpea Spread

Makes 4 cups

Chickpeas and orange provide antioxidants, while tuna supplies healthy fat. Serve this smooth, hummus-like spread with fresh vegetable sticks as a dipper, or slather on whole-grain crackers or toast. If you can't find white balsamic vinegar, go with the darker variety. Just know that it will affect the color of the dip.

1 pound low-mercury, BPA-free canned tuna
1 cup rinsed and drained canned (BPA-free) chickpeas
6 tablespoons extra-virgin olive oil
¼ cup fresh orange juice
¼ cup white balsamic vinegar
2 tablespoons fresh rosemary leaves (from about 2 sprigs)
½ teaspoon salt
¼ teaspoon black pepper

Add all of the ingredients to a food processor, and puree until smooth.

◆ ◆ ◆

Carrot-Miso Dressing

Makes 1½ cups

With miso, orange juice, and carrot, this brightly hued salad dressing or dip is full of prostate-friendly antioxidants. Garlic and ginger have also been shown to have health-protective effects. Toss with greens or serve with fresh vegetable sticks. Or convert into a meal: toss with salad greens, then top with roasted salmon, tofu, or chicken.

One 1-inch-square piece peeled fresh ginger root
1 medium garlic clove

1 cup thinly sliced peeled carrot
¼ cup plus 2 tablespoons avocado oil
¼ cup unseasoned rice vinegar
3 tablespoons fresh orange juice
2 tablespoons mirin (Japanese rice wine)
2 tablespoons miso paste
2 teaspoons honey
½ teaspoon salt

Add the ginger and garlic to a food processor and process until minced, about 10 seconds. Add the remaining ingredients and puree until smooth.

◆ ◆ ◆

Chunky Spiced Pear Sauce

Makes about 2¾ cups

Serve this naturally sweet sauce over oatmeal, pancakes, or plant-based yogurt. Top with toasted nuts. For variety, you can also use sweet apples (such as Honeycrisp or Pink Lady) or even frozen sweet fruit, like cherries, mango, or pineapple.

3 large, extremely ripe sweet pears, such as Comice, unpeeled
    and chopped (about 5 cups)
Scant ¼ cup fresh orange juice
½ teaspoon salt
½ teaspoon ground cardamom or cinnamon

Add all the ingredients to a medium pot, and bring to a boil over high heat.

Once boiling, cover and reduce heat to medium-low. Simmer for 15 minutes.

Mash with a potato masher and increase heat to high. Boil for another 5 minutes.

METRIC CONVERSION CHART

Useful Equivalents for Dry Ingredients by Weight
(To convert ounces to grams, multiply the number of ounces by 30.)

1 oz	1/16 lb	30 g
4 oz	¼ lb	120 g
8 oz	½ lb	240 g
12 oz	¾ lb	360 g
16 oz	1 lb	480 g

Useful Equivalents for Cooking/Oven Temperatures

Process	Fahrenheit	Celsius	Gas Mark
Freeze Water	32° F	0° C	
Room Temperature	68° F	20° C	
Boil Water	212° F	100° C	
Bake	325° F	160° C	3
	350° F	180° C	4
	375° F	190° C	5
	400° F	200° C	6
	425° F	220° C	7
	450° F	230° C	8
Broil			Grill

Useful Equivalents for Length
(To convert inches to centimeters, multiply the number of inches by 2.5.)

1 in			2.5 cm	
6 in	½ ft		15 cm	
12 in	1 ft		30 cm	
36 in	3 ft	1 yd	90 cm	
40 in			100 cm	1 m

GLOSSARY

active surveillance: This involves delayed treatment. The patient is closely supervised by medical professionals but not given treatment unless the condition worsens. This approach is an option when prostate cancer is low-risk and the patient wants to avoid potential side effects of treatment. This is different than the term "watchful waiting."

adrenal glands: Glands located on top of both kidneys that produce important hormones that modulate the stress response, blood sugar control, immune response, and other processes. Examples of adrenal hormones include DHEA, cortisol, pregnenolone, epinephrine, and norepinephrine.

andropause: A decline of testosterone levels and signs and symptoms associated with reduction in this hormone. Andropause normally starts in middle-aged men.

aromatase: An enzyme that converts testosterone into estrogen.

benign prostatic hyperplasia (BPH): An age-associated condition that involves enlargement of the prostate gland.

bioidentical hormone replacement: Hormone therapy that involves hormones that have the same structure and function as those produced by the human body. Oppositely, synthetic hormones would be altered such that they are not identical to the structure and function of hormones as found in the human body.

bulbourethral glands: A pair of glands located beneath the prostate in males. They function to secrete fluid that supports semen flow and fertility.

chronic pelvic pain syndrome (CPPS): Unexplained chronic pelvic pain in men when there is no detectable infection. It involves pain associated with urination and/or pain in the groin, genitalia, or perineum (the area between the anus and scrotum).

complementary and alternative medicine (CAM): Treatments such as nutrition, herbs, vitamins, minerals, dietary supplements, and other holistic, nondrug therapies as an addition to standard medical treatments. Also referred to as integrative medicine.

dehydroepiandrosterone (DHEA): A steroidal hormone that is produced mainly by the adrenal glands and in small amounts by the ovaries, testes, and brain. It has direct effects on cells in the body and is a precursor hormone for the production of estradiol and testosterone.

dihydrotestosterone (DHT): A metabolite of testosterone that stimulates prostate gland growth.

dysuria: Difficulty or pain with urination.

endocrine-disrupting chemicals (EDCs): Generally, this refers to human-made chemicals that interfere with the synthesis and action of hormones.

erectile dysfunction (ED): The inability to get or keep an erection for sexual intercourse.

estrogen: A hormone produced in both females and males. In males it is produced in fat and bone and by the conversion of the hormone androstenedione into estrogen.

5-alpha-reductase: An enzyme that converts testosterone into DHT. Medications used to inhibit this conversion are known as 5-alpha-reductase inhibitors (5-ARIs). They are used to treat BPH.

follicle-stimulating hormone (FSH): A hormone produced by the anterior pituitary gland that stimulates the Sertoli cells of the testes to produce sperm.

Gleason score: The grading of prostate cancer according to the appearance of prostate cells that have been biopsied and analyzed. A newer system developed by the International Society of Urological Pathologists created a supplementary guide called the Grade Groups.

gonadotropin-releasing hormone (GnRH): A hormone produced and released by the hypothalamus region of the brain. GnRH stimulates the release of FSH and LH by the pituitary gland, which ultimately results in sperm and testosterone production by the testes.

hormone replacement: The administration of hormones as a treatment for hormone deficiencies.

hypogonadism: A deficiency of testosterone production by the testes.

hypothalamus: An area of the brain that produces hormones that stimulate pituitary hormones such as FSH and LH to be released.

integrative medicine: A medical approach that takes into account the whole person. This system of medicine seeks to treat root causes of a person's health problems. Therapies can involve conventional and holistic approaches.

International Prostate Symptom Score (IPSS): A questionnaire used to assess the severity of lower urinary tract symptoms associated with BPH.

Leydig cells: Specialized cells in the testes that produce testosterone.

libido: Sex drive.

lower urinary tract symptoms (LUTS): Symptoms related to problems of the lower urinary tract, which includes the bladder, prostate, and urethra.

luteinizing hormone (LH): A hormone produced by the anterior pituitary gland that stimulates the testes to produce testosterone.

Mediterranean diet: A diet consisting of plenty of plant foods (fruits, vegetables, legumes, nuts, breads, and unrefined cereals); lots of olive oil; moderately high intake of fish; moderate consumption of alcohol; and low consumption of poultry, red meat, and eggs.

nocturia: Nighttime urination. This is common with BPH and urinary incontinence.

pelvic floor: Muscles in the floor of the pelvis that support organs in the region.

phosphodiesterase-5 inhibitors (PDE5 inhibitors): Commonly used medications for the treatment of erectile dysfunction (ED).

polyphenols: A category of plant compounds found in a number of plant-based foods that have several health benefits.

prostate cancer: Malignant growths (cancer) that occur in the prostate.

prostate gland: A male gland located beneath the bladder and in front of the rectum. The prostate functions to produce fluid that nourishes and protects sperm, which is essential for fertility.

prostate-specific antigen (PSA): This protein is produced by the prostate and functions to aid sperm fertility. Elevated blood levels of PSA are associated with BPH, prostatitis, and prostate cancer.

prostatitis: Inflammation and/or infection of the prostate gland. This condition can be acute or chronic.

seminiferous tubules: Specialized tubules that produce, store, and mature sperm in each testicle.

Sertoli cells: Specialized cells that manufacture sperm in the testes.

sex hormone–binding globulin (SHBG): A protein carrier of the hormones testosterone and estradiol.

testes: Plural word for the testicles.

testicle: The male reproductive organ that produces sperm and testosterone. One testicle is referred to as a testis.

testosterone: A hormone produced by the Leydig cells of the testes that has several functions in the male body.

xenoestrogens: Chemicals in the environment that mimic human estrogen. As a result, they can disrupt estrogen balance in the body.

watchful waiting: An approach used by older men with prostate cancer (or other cancers) who are expected to live less than five years and who decline conventional therapies unless symptoms appear or change.

ENDNOTES

Chapter 1: Healing the Prostate—
Why Every Man Must Take Action

1. Levi A. Deters et al., "How Common Is Benign Prostatic Hyperplasia (BPH)?" Medscape, January 15, 2019, https://www.medscape.com/answers/437359-90389/how-common-is-benign-prostatic-hyperplasia-bph.

2. "Key Statistics for Prostate Cancer," Cancer.org, January 8, 2020, https://www.cancer.org/cancer/prostate-cancer/about/key-statistics.html.

3. "Key Statistics," Cancer.org.

4. "Prostatitis: Inflammation of the Prostate," NIDDK, July 2014, https://www.niddk.nih.gov/health-information/urologic-diseases/prostate-problems/prostatitis-inflammation-prostate.

5. "Low Testosterone (Low T): Causes, Symptoms, Diagnosis & Treatment," Cleveland Clinic, 2020, https://my.clevelandclinic.org/health/diseases/15603-low-testosterone-male-hypogonadism.

6. Chun-Hou Liao and Hann-Chorng Kuo, "Measurement of International Prostate Symptom Score Subscores in Male Lower Urinary Tract Symptoms," *Incontinence of Pelvic Floor Dysfunction* 4, no. 2 (2010): 39–43.

7. Nazia Q. Bandukwala, "Men with Incontinence: Treating and Managing," WebMD, September 17, 2019, https://www.webmd.com/urinary-incontinence-oab/ss/slideshow-male-incontinence.

8. Nicolas A. Muruve, "Prostate Anatomy," Medscape, September 13, 2017, https://emedicine.medscape.com/article/1923122-overview.

9. Claus Roehrborn, "What We Know about Your Prostate," UT Southwestern Medical Center, November 9, 2018, https://utswmed.org/medblog/what-we-know-about-your-prostate.

10. Jerry Bergman, *Poor Design: An Invalid Argument against Intelligent Design* (Tulsa: BP Books, 2019).

11. Muruve, "Prostate Anatomy."

12. Muruve, "Prostate Anatomy."

13. "Prostate Cancer," Canadian Cancer Society, https://www.cancer
.ca/en/cancer-information/cancer-type/prostate/prostate-cancer
/the-prostate/?region=on.

14. "Prostate Cancer," Canadian Cancer Society.

15. John E. Hall, *Guyton and Hall Textbook of Medical Physiology,* 13th
ed. reprint, Kindle edition (London: Elsevier Health Sciences,
2016).

16. Hall, *Textbook of Medical Physiology.*

17. Hall, *Textbook of Medical Physiology.*

18. Hall, *Textbook of Medical Physiology.*

19. Nishi Gupta et al., "Mutations in the Prostate Specific Antigen
(PSA/KLK3) Correlate with Male Infertility," *Scientific Reports* 7, no.
1 (2017), doi: 10.1038/s41598-017-10866-1.

20. John E. Hall, *Guyton and Hall Textbook of Medical Physiology,* 13th
ed. reprint, Kindle edition (London: Elsevier Health Sciences:
2016).

21. Richard A. Watson, "Chronic Pelvic Pain in Men: Practice
Essentials, Etiology, Epidemiology," Medscape, March 17, 2020,
https://emedicine.medscape.com/article/437745-overview.

22. Prashanth Rawla, "Epidemiology of Prostate Cancer," *World Journal
of Oncology* 10, no. 2 (2019): 63–89, doi: 10.14740/wjon1191.

23. Gerald R. Cunha et al., "Development of the Human Prostate,"
Differentiation 103 (2018), doi: 10.1016/j.diff.2018.08.005.

24. Cunha et al., "Development of the Human Prostate."

25. Cunha et al., "Development of the Human Prostate."

26. K. Das and N. Buchholz, "Benign Prostate Hyperplasia and
Nutrition," *Clinical Nutrition ESPEN* 33 (2019): 5–11, doi: 10.1016
/j.clnesp.2019.07.015.

27. E. W. Rugendorff et al., "Results of Treatment with Pollen Extract
(Cernilton N) in Chronic Prostatitis and Prostatodynia," *British
Journal of Urology* 71, no. 4 (1993): 433–38, doi: 10.1111
/j.1464-410x.1993.tb15988.x.

28. Dean Ornish et al., "Intensive Lifestyle Changes May Affect the
Progression of Prostate Cancer," *Journal of Urology* 174, no. 3 (2005):
1065–70, doi: 10.1097/01.ju.0000169487.49018.73.

29. Niikee Schoendorfer et al., "Urox Containing Concentrated Extracts of *Crataeva nurvala* Stem Bark, *Equisetum arvense* Stem and *Lindera aggregata* Root, in the Treatment of Symptoms of Overactive Bladder and Urinary Incontinence: A Phase 2, Randomised, Double-Blind Placebo Controlled Trial," *BMC Complementary and Alternative Medicine* 18, no. 1 (2018), doi: 10.1186/s12906 -018-2101-4.

Chapter 2: Prostate Enlargement (BPH) Causes and Solutions

1. "Prostate Enlargement (Benign Prostatic Hyperplasia)," NIDDK, September 2014, https://www.niddk.nih.gov/health-information /urologic-diseases/prostate-problems/prostate-enlargement -benign-prostatic-hyperplasia.

2. Levi A. Deters et al., "Benign Prostatic Hyperplasia (BPH): Practice Essentials, Background, Anatomy," Medscape, January 15, 2019, https://emedicine.medscape.com/article/437359-overview.

3. Deters et al., "Practice Essentials."

4. *Benign Prostatic Hyperplasia (BPH) Patient Guide*, e-book (Linthicum: Urology Care Foundation, 2020), http://www.urologyhealth.org.

5. "Prostate Enlargement," NIDDK.

6. Marcello Henrique Araujo Da Silva and Diogo Benchimol De Souza, "Current Evidence for the Involvement of Sex Steroid Receptors and Sex Hormones in Benign Prostatic Hyperplasia," *Research and Reports in Urology* 11 (2019): 1–8, doi: 10.2147/rru.s155609.

7. Deters et al., "Practice Essentials."

8. Da Silva and De Souza, "Current Evidence."

9. Da Silva and De Souza, "Current Evidence."

10. Da Silva and De Souza, "Current Evidence."

11. Da Silva and De Souza, "Current Evidence."

12. Paul G. Cohen, "Obesity in Men: The Hypogonadal–Estrogen Receptor Relationship and Its Effect on Glucose Homeostasis," *Medical Hypotheses* 70, no. 2 (2008): 358–60, doi: 10.1016 /j.mehy.2007.05.020.

13. Domenico Prezioso et al., "Estrogens and Aspects of Prostate Disease," *International Journal of Urology* 14, no. 1 (2006): 1–16, doi: 10.1111/j.1442-2042.2006.01476.x.

14. Prezioso et al., "Estrogens and Aspects."

15. Da Silva and De Souza, "Current Evidence."

16. Da Silva and De Souza, "Current Evidence."

17. Thea Grindstad et al., "Progesterone Receptors in Prostate Cancer: Progesterone Receptor B Is the Isoform Associated with Disease Progression," *Scientific Reports* 8, no. 1 (2018), doi: 10.1038 /s41598-018-29520-5.

18. Deters et al., "Practice Essentials."

19. K. Das and N. Buchholz, "Benign Prostate Hyperplasia and Nutrition," *Clinical Nutrition ESPEN* 33 (2019): 5–11, doi: 10.1016 /j.clnesp.2019.07.015.

20. Das and Buchholz, "Benign Prostate Hyperplasia and Nutrition."

21. *Benign Prostatic Hyperplasia (BPH) Patient Guide*, e-book (Linthicum: Urology Care Foundation, 2020), http://www.urologyhealth.org.

22. *Benign Prostatic Hyperplasia (BPH) Patient Guide.*

23. "Benign Prostatic Hyperplasia (BPH): Symptoms, Diagnosis & Treatment," Urology Care Foundation, August 2020, https://www.urologyhealth.org/urologic-conditions /benign-prostatic-hyperplasia-(bph).

24. "Benign Prostatic Hyperplasia (BPH)," Urology Care Foundation.

25. "Benign Prostatic Hyperplasia (BPH)," Urology Care Foundation.

26. "Benign Prostatic Hyperplasia (BPH)," Johns Hopkins Medicine, https://www.hopkinsmedicine.org/health/conditions-and-diseases /benign-prostatic-hyperplasia-bph.

27. "Benign Prostatic Hyperplasia (BPH)," Johns Hopkins Medicine.

28. "Benign Prostatic Hyperplasia (BPH)," Johns Hopkins Medicine.

29. Da Silva and De Souza, "Current Evidence."

30. Da Silva and De Souza, "Current Evidence."

31. "Prostate Enlargement," NIDDK.

32. "Prostate Enlargement," NIDDK.

33. "Prostate Enlargement," NIDDK.

34. Levi A. Deters et al., "Which Medications in the Drug Class Alpha-Adrenergic Blockers Are Used in the Treatment of Benign Prostatic Hyperplasia (BPH)?" Medscape, January 15, 2019, https:// emedicine.medscape.com/article/437359-questions-and-answers.

35. Manasi Jiwrajka et al., "Drugs for Benign Prostatic Hypertrophy," *Australian Prescriber* 41, no. 5 (2018): 150–53, doi: 10.18773 /austprescr.2018.045.

36. Leigh Anderson, "Benign Prostatic Hypertrophy (BPH): Symptoms and Treatment," Drugs.com, April 23, 2019, https://www.drugs.com /article/benign-prostatic-hypertrophy.html.

37. Philipp Dahm et al., "Comparative Effectiveness of Newer Medications for Lower Urinary Tract Symptoms Attributed to Benign Prostatic Hyperplasia: A Systematic Review and Meta-Analysis," *European Urology* 71, no. 4 (2017): 570–81, doi: 10.1016 /j.eururo.2016.09.032.

38. Dahm et al., "Comparative Effectiveness."

39. Dahm et al., "Comparative Effectiveness."

40. Anderson, "Symptoms and Treatment"; and Jiwrajka et al., "Drugs for Benign Prostatic Hypertrophy."

41. Levi A. Deters et al., "Benign Prostatic Hyperplasia (BPH) Medication," Medscape, January 15, 2019, https://emedicine .medscape.com/article/437359-medication.

42. Eric H. Kim, John A. Brockman, and Gerald L. Andriole, "The Use of 5-Alpha Reductase Inhibitors in the Treatment of Benign Prostatic Hyperplasia," *Asian Journal of Urology* 5, no. 1 (2018): 28–32, doi: 10.1016/j.ajur.2017.11.005.

43. "Prostate Enlargement," NIDDK.

44. Jiwrajka et al., "Drugs for Benign Prostatic Hypertrophy."

45. Anderson, "Symptoms and Treatment."

46. "Prostate Enlargement," NIDDK.

47. Anderson, "Symptoms and Treatment."

48. Jiwrajka et al., "Drugs for Benign Prostatic Hypertrophy."

49. Michael A. Liss and Ian M. Thompson, "Prostate Cancer Prevention with 5-Alpha Reductase Inhibitors," *Current Opinion in Urology* 28, no. 1 (2018): 42–45, doi: 10.1097/mou.0000000000000464.

50. Liss and Thompson, "Prostate Cancer Prevention."

51. Deters et al., "Benign Prostatic Hyperplasia (BPH) Medication."

52. Jiwrajka et al., "Drugs for Benign Prostatic Hypertrophy."

53. Jiwrajka et al., "Drugs for Benign Prostatic Hypertrophy."

54. "Tadalafil (Rx)," Medscape, https://reference.medscape.com /drug/adcirca-cialis-tadalafil-342873.

55. "Tadalafil (Rx)," Medscape.

56. "Tadalafil (Rx)," Medscape.

57. "Benign Prostatic Hyperplasia (BPH)," Urology Care Foundation.

58. Omer A. Raheem and J. Kellogg Parsons, "Associations of Obesity, Physical Activity and Diet with Benign Prostatic Hyperplasia and Lower Urinary Tract Symptoms," *Current Opinion in Urology* 24, no. 1 (2014): 10–14, doi: 10.1097/mou.0000000000000004.

59. Das and Buchholz, "Benign Prostate Hyperplasia and Nutrition."

60. Kathleen Y. Wolin et al., "Physical Activity and Benign Prostatic Hyperplasia-Related Outcomes and Nocturia," *Medicine & Science in Sports & Exercise* 47, no. 3 (2015): 581–92, doi: 10.1249 /mss.0000000000000444.

61. Ji Hwan Kim, Kyung Moo Park, and Ju Ah Lee, "Herbal Medicine for Benign Prostatic Hyperplasia," *Medicine* 98, no. 1 (2019): e14023, doi: 10.1097/md.0000000000014023.

62. Geovanni Espinosa and Michael T. Murray, "Benign Prostatic Hyperplasia," in *Textbook of Natural Medicine*, eds. Michael T. Murray and Joseph E. Pizzorno, 4th ed. reprint (St. Louis, MO: Churchill Livingstone, 2013), 1266.

63. Brett Lomenick et al., "Identification and Characterization of Beta-Sitosterol Target Proteins," *Bioorganic & Medicinal Chemistry Letters* 25, no. 21 (2015): 4976–79, doi: 10.1016/j.bmcl.2015.03.007.

64. Timothy J. Wilt et al., "Beta-Sitosterols for Benign Prostatic Hyperplasia," *Cochrane Database of Systematic Reviews*, July 26, 1999, doi: 10.1002/14651858.cd001043.

65. R. R. Berges et al., "Randomised, Placebo-Controlled, Double-Blind Clinical Trial of Beta-Sitosterol in Patients with Benign Prostatic Hyperplasia," *The Lancet* 345, no. 8964 (1995): 1529–32, doi: 10.1016/s0140-6736(95)91085-9.

66. K. F. Klippel, D. M. Hiltl, and B. Schipp, "A Multicentric, Placebo-Controlled, Double-Blind Clinical Trial of Beta-Sitosterol (Phytosterol) for the Treatment of Benign Prostatic Hyperplasia," *BJU International* 80, no. 3 (1997): 427–32, doi: 10.1046 /j.1464-410x.1997.t01-1-00362.x.

67. Wilt et al., "Beta-Sitosterols."

68. Nishtman Dizeyi et al., "The Effects of Cernitin® on Inflammatory Parameters and Benign Prostatic Hyperplasia: An In Vitro Study," *Phytotherapy Research* 33, no. 9 (2019): 2457–64, doi: 10.1002 /ptr.6438.

69. Ryoji Yasumoto et al., "Clinical Evaluation of Long-Term Treatment Using Cernitin Pollen Extract in Patients with Benign Prostatic Hyperplasia," *Clinical Therapeutics* 17, no. 1 (1995): 82–87, doi: 10.1016/0149-2918(95)80009-3.

70. Harry G. Preuss et al., "Randomized Trial of a Combination of Natural Products (Cernitin, Saw Palmetto, B-Sitosterol, Vitamin E) on Symptoms of Benign Prostatic Hyperplasia (BPH),"

International Urology and Nephrology 33, no. 2 (2001): 217–25, doi: 10.1023/a:1015227604041.

71. Stephen Bent et al., "Saw Palmetto for Benign Prostatic Hyperplasia," *New England Journal of Medicine* 354, no. 6 (2006): 557–66, doi: 10.1056/nejmoa053085.

72. Eric L. Yarnell and Kathy Abascal, "*Serenoa repens* (Saw Palmetto)," in *Textbook of Natural Medicine*, eds. Michael T. Murray and Joseph E. Pizzorno, 4th ed. reprint (St. Louis, MO: Churchill Livingstone, 2013), 1267.

73. Espinosa and Murray, "Benign Prostatic Hyperplasia."

74. Remigio Vela-Navarrete et al., "Efficacy and Safety of a Hexanic Extract of *Serenoa repens* (Permixon®) for the Treatment of Lower Urinary Tract Symptoms Associated with Benign Prostatic Hyperplasia (LUTS/BPH): Systematic Review and Meta-Analysis of Randomised Controlled Trials and Observational Studies," *BJU International* 122, no. 6 (2018): 1049–65, doi: 10.1111/bju.14362.

75. Timothy J. Wilt, Areef Ishani, and Roderick MacDonald, "*Serenoa repens* for Benign Prostatic Hyperplasia," *Cochrane Database of Systematic Reviews*, July 22, 2002, doi: 10.1002/14651858.cd001423.

76. Michael J. Barry et al., "Effect of Increasing Doses of Saw Palmetto Extract on Lower Urinary Tract Symptoms," *JAMA* 306, no. 12 (2011): 1344–51, doi: 10.1001/jama.2011.1364; and Bent et al., "Saw Palmetto."

77. Espinosa and Murray, "Benign Prostatic Hyperplasia."

78. Jason Ricco and Shailendra Prasad, "PURLs: The Shrinking Case for Saw Palmetto," *The Journal of Family Practice* 61, no. 7 (2012): 418–20.

79. Vela-Navarrete et al., "Efficacy and Safety."

80. Youngjoo Kwon, "Use of Saw Palmetto (*Serenoa repens*) Extract for Benign Prostatic Hyperplasia," *Food Science and Biotechnology* 28, no. 6 (2019): 1599–1606, doi: 10.1007/s10068-019-00605-9.

81. Nikolai Lopatkin et al., "Efficacy and Safety of a Combination of Sabal and Urtica Extract in Lower Urinary Tract Symptoms— Long-Term Follow-Up of a Placebo-Controlled, Double-Blind, Multicenter Trial," *International Urology and Nephrology* 39, no. 4 (2007): 1137–46, doi: 10.1007/s11255-006-9173-7.

82. T. B. Agbabiaka et al., "*Serenoa repens* (Saw Palmetto): A Systematic Review of Adverse Events," *Drug-Safety* 32, no. 8 (2009): 637–47, https://www.ncbi.nlm.nih.gov/books/NBK76603.

83. Michael T. Murray, "*Pygeum africanum* (Bitter Almond)," in *Textbook of Natural Medicine*, eds. Michael T. Murray and Joseph E. Pizzorno, 4th ed. reprint (St. Louis, MO: Churchill Livingstone, 2013), 1002; and Espinosa and Murray, "Benign Prostatic Hyperplasia."

84. Murray, "*Pygeum africanum*."

85. Murray, "*Pygeum africanum*."

86. Maria T. Quiles et al., "Antiproliferative and Apoptotic Effects of the Herbal Agent *Pygeum africanum* on Cultured Prostate Stromal Cells from Patients with Benign Prostatic Hyperplasia (BPH)," *The Prostate* 70, no. 10 (2010): 1044–53, doi: 10.1002/pros.21138.

87. J. Salinas-Casado et al., "Revisión sobre la Experiencia y Evidencias del *Pygeum africanum* en Urología," *Actas Urológicas Españolas* 44, no. 1 (2020): 9–13, doi: 10.1016/j.acuro.2019.08.002.

88. Timothy Wilt and Areef Ishani, "*Pygeum africanum* for Benign Prostatic Hyperplasia," *Cochrane Database of Systematic Reviews*, January 26, 1998, doi: 10.1002/14651858.cd001044.

89. C. Chatelain, W. Autet, and F. Brackman, "Comparison of Once and Twice Daily Dosage Forms of *Pygeum africanum* Extract in Patients with Benign Prostatic Hyperplasia: A Randomized, Double-Blind Study, with Long-Term Open Label Extension," *Urology* 54, no. 3 (1999): 473–78, doi: 10.1016/s0090-4295(99)00147-8.

90. J. Salinas-Casado et al., *Actas Urológicas Españolas*.

91. Wilt and Ishani, "*Pygeum africanum*."

92. Julia E. Chrubasik et al., "A Comprehensive Review on the Stinging Nettle Effect and Efficacy Profiles. Part II: *Urticae radix*," *Phytomedicine* 14, nos. 7–8 (2007): 568–79, doi: 10.1016/j.phymed.2007.03.014.

93. Mohammad Reza Safarinejad, "*Urtica dioica* for Treatment of Benign Prostatic Hyperplasia: A Prospective, Randomized, Double-Blind, Placebo-Controlled, Crossover Study," *Journal of Herbal Pharmacotherapy* 5, no. 4 (2005): 1–11, doi: 10.1080/J157v05n04_01.

94. Alireza Ghorbanibirgani, Ali Khalili, and Laleh Zamani, "The Efficacy of Stinging Nettle (*Urtica dioica*) in Patients with Benign Prostatic Hyperplasia: A Randomized Double-Blind Study in 100 Patients," *Iranian Red Crescent Medical Journal* 15, no. 1 (2013), doi: 10.5812/ircmj.2386.

95. Lopatkin et al., "Efficacy and Safety of a Combination of Sabal and Urtica Extract in Lower Urinary Tract Symptoms."

96. Boris Bondarenko et al., "Long-Term Efficacy and Safety of PRO 160/120 (A Combination of Sabal and Urtica Extract) in Patients with Lower Urinary Tract Symptoms (LUTS)," *Phytomedicine* 10 (2003): 53–55, doi: 10.1078/1433-187x-00352.

97. Andrea Ledda et al., "Benign Prostatic Hypertrophy: Pycnogenol® Supplementation Improves Prostate Symptoms and Residual Bladder Volume," *Minerva Medica* 109, no. 4 (2018): 280–84, doi: 10.23736/S0026-4806.18.05572-6.

98. Abeer M. Mahmoud et al., "Zinc Intake and Risk of Prostate Cancer: Case-Control Study and Meta-Analysis," *PLOS ONE* 11, no. 11 (2016): e0165956, doi: 10.1371/journal.pone.0165956.

99. Alan R. Kristal et al., "Dietary Patterns, Supplement Use, and the Risk of Symptomatic Benign Prostatic Hyperplasia: Results from the Prostate Cancer Prevention Trial," *American Journal of Epidemiology* 167, no. 8 (2008): 925–34, doi: 10.1093/aje/kwm389.

100. Pamela Christudoss et al., "Zinc Status of Patients with Benign Prostatic Hyperplasia and Prostate Carcinoma," *Indian Journal of Urology* 27, no. 1 (2011): 14–18, doi: 10.4103/0970-1591.78405.

101. Jane Higdon et al., "Zinc," Linus Pauling Institute, May 2019, https://lpi.oregonstate.edu/mic/minerals/zinc.

102. Higdon et al., "Zinc."

103. Mohamed Abdemonem Elshazly et al., "Vitamin D Deficiency and Lower Urinary Tract Symptoms in Males above 50 Years of Age," *Urology Annals* 9, no. 2 (2017): 170–73, doi: 10.4103/0974-7796.204192.

104. Camille P. Vaughan et al., "Vitamin D and Lower Urinary Tract Symptoms among US Men: Results from the 2005–2006 National Health and Nutrition Examination Survey," *Urology* 78, no. 6 (2011): 1292–97, doi: 10.1016/j.urology.2011.07.1415.

105. Vaughan et al., "Vitamin D."

106. Yoon Jung Yang et al., "Comparison of Fatty Acid Profiles in the Serum of Patients with Prostate Cancer and Benign Prostatic Hyperplasia," *Clinical Biochemistry* 32, no. 6 (1999): 405–9, doi: 10.1016/s0009-9120(99)00036-3.

107. Alireza Ghadian and Mehran Rezaei, "Combination Therapy with Omega-3 Fatty Acids Plus Tamsulocin and Finasteride in the Treatment of Men with Lower Urinary Tract Symptoms (LUTS) and Benign Prostatic Hyperplasia (BPH)," *Inflammopharmacology* 25, no. 4 (2017): 451–58, doi: 10.1007/s10787-017-0343-2.

108. Kim, Park, and Lee, "Herbal Medicine for Benign Prostatic Hyperplasia."

109. Wei Zhang et al., "Acupuncture for Benign Prostatic Hyperplasia: A Systematic Review and Meta-Analysis," *PLOS ONE* 12, no. 4 (2017): e0174586, doi: 10.1371/journal.pone.0174586.

Chapter 3: The Bladder Factor for BPH and Urinary Control

1. S. Siracusano et al., "Catheters and Infections," in *Clinical Management of Complicated Urinary Tract Infection*, ed. Ahmad Nikibakhsh, IntechOpen, September 6, 2011, doi: 10.5772/21877.

2. Siracusano et al., "Catheters and Infections."

3. Chun-Hou Liao and Hann-Chorng Kuo, "Measurement of International Prostate Symptom Score Subscores in Male Lower Urinary Tract Symptoms," *Incontinence of Pelvic Floor Dysfunction* 4, no. 2 (2010): 39–43.

4. Hann-Chorng Kuo, "Male Lower Urinary Tract Symptoms: An Old Problem from a New Perspective," *Incontinence Pelvic Floor Dysfunction* 4, no. 2 (2010): 33–38.

5. Liao and Kuo, "International Prostate Symptom Score Subscores."

6. Liao and Kuo, "International Prostate Symptom Score Subscores."

7. Liao and Kuo, "International Prostate Symptom Score Subscores."

8. Wellman W. Cheung et al., "Prevalence, Evaluation and Management of Overactive Bladder in Primary Care," *BMC Family Practice* 10, no. 1 (2009), doi: 10.1186/1471-2296-10-8.

9. Roger Blackmore, "ICS Fact Sheets 2015," International Continence Society, September 4, 2015, https://www.ics.org; and Kuo, "Male Lower Urinary Tract Symptoms."

10. Blackmore, "ICS Fact Sheets 2015"; and Kuo, "Male Lower Urinary Tract Symptoms."

11. "Overactive Bladder (OAB): Symptoms, Diagnosis & Treatment," Urology Care Foundation, https://www.urologyhealth.org /urologic-conditions/overactive-bladder-(oab).

12. "Overactive Bladder (OAB)," Urology Care Foundation.

13. Blackmore, "ICS Fact Sheets 2015."

14. "Overactive Bladder (OAB)," Urology Care Foundation; and Pamela I. Ellsworth, "What Is the Role of Medications in Treating Overactive Bladder?" MedicineNet, https://www.medicinenet.com /overactive_bladder/article.htm.

15. Ellsworth, "What Is the Role of Medications?"

16. Omudhome Ogbru, "Mirabegron," MedicineNet, https://www .medicinenet.com/mirabegron/article.htm.

17. Pamela I. Ellsworth, "Overactive Bladder Medication," Medscape, January 27, 2020, https://emedicine.medscape.com/article /459340-medication#5.

18. Shelly L. Gray et al., "Cumulative Use of Strong Anticholinergics and Incident Dementia," *JAMA Internal Medicine* 175, no. 3 (2015): 401–7, doi: 10.1001/jamainternmed.2014.7663.

19. Jamie Santa Cruz, "Botox as Incontinence Therapy," Today's Geriatric Medicine, https://www.todaysgeriatricmedicine.com /news/ex_100615.shtml.

20. "Urinary Incontinence in Men," MedicineNet, https://www .medicinenet.com/urinary_incontinence/article.htm.

21. "Incontinence: Symptoms & Treatment," Urology Care Foundation, April 2020, https://www.urologyhealth.org /urologic-conditions/urinary-incontinence.

22. Sandip P. Vasavada, Maude E. Carmel, and Raymond R. Rackley, "Urinary Incontinence: Practice Essentials, Background, Anatomy," Medscape, September 23, 2019, https://emedicine.medscape.com /article/452289-overview.

23. Vasavada, Carmel, and Rackley, "Urinary Incontinence."

24. Niikee Schoendorfer et al., "Urox Containing Concentrated Extracts of *Crataeva nurvala* Stem Bark, *Equisetum arvense* Stem and *Lindera aggregata* Root, in the Treatment of Symptoms of Overactive Bladder and Urinary Incontinence: A Phase 2, Randomised, Double-Blind Placebo Controlled Trial," *BMC Complementary and Alternative Medicine* 18, no. 1 (2018), doi: 10.1186/s12906-018-2101-4.

25. Schoendorfer et al., "Urox Containing Concentrated Extracts."

26. Ali Esmail Al-Snafi, "The Pharmacology of *Equisetum arvense*: A Review," *IOSR Journal of Pharmacy (IOSRPHR)* 7, no. 2 (2017): 31–42, doi: 10.9790/3013-0702013142.

27. Schoendorfer et al., "Urox Containing Concentrated Extracts."

28. Schoendorfer et al., "Urox Containing Concentrated Extracts."

29. Schoendorfer et al., "Urox Containing Concentrated Extracts."

30. Mie Nishimura et al., "Pumpkin Seed Oil Extracted from *Cucurbita maxima* Improves Urinary Disorder in Human Overactive Bladder," *Journal of Traditional and Complementary Medicine* 4, no. 1 (2014): 72–74, doi: 10.4103/2225-4110.124355.

31. M. Friederich, C. Theurer, and G. Schiebel-Schlosser, "Prosta Fink Forte®-Kapseln in der Behandlung der benignen Prostatahyperplasie. Eine multizentrische Anwendungsbeobachtung an 2245 Patienten," *Complementary Medicine Research* 7, no. 4 (2000): 200–04, doi: 10.1159/000021344.

32. Bongseok Shim et al., "A Randomized Double-Blind Placebo-Controlled Clinical Trial of a Product Containing Pumpkin Seed Extract and Soy Germ Extract to Improve Overactive Bladder-Related Voiding Dysfunction and Quality of Life," *Journal of Functional Foods* 8 (2014): 111–17, doi: 10.1016/j.jff.2014.03.010.

33. Ales Vidlar et al., "Cranberry Fruit Powder (Flowens™) Improves Lower Urinary Tract Symptoms in Men: A Double-Blind, Randomized, Placebo-Controlled Study," *World Journal of Urology* 34, no. 3 (2015): 419–24, doi: 10.1007/s00345-015-1611-7.

34. Ales Vidlar. et al., "The Effectiveness of Dried Cranberries (*Vaccinium macrocarpon*) in Men with Lower Urinary Tract Symptoms," *British Journal of Nutrition* 104, no. 8 (2010): 1181–89, doi: 10.1017/S0007114510002059.

35. Jennifer K. Nelson, "Are There Dietary Changes I Can Make to Deal with Overactive Bladder?" Mayo Clinic, April 17, 2020, https://www.mayoclinic.org/healthy-lifestyle/nutrition-and-healthy-eating/expert-answers/diet-and-overactive-bladder/faq-20322774; and "Overactive Bladder (OAB)," Urology Care Foundation.

36. Mohsen Khamessipour and Michael Hall, "The Effects of Chiropractic Spinal Manipulation on Urinary Incontinence in Patients with Low Back Pain and Radiculopathy: A Retrospective Case Series Report," *Journal of Alternative, Complementary & Integrative Medicine* 3, no. 4 (2017): 1–7, doi: 10.24966/ACIM-7562/100042.

37. Yuwei Zhao et al., "Acupuncture for Adults with Overactive Bladder," *Medicine (Baltimore)* 97, no. 8 (2018): e9838, doi: 10.1097/MD.0000000000009838.

Chapter 4: Prostatitis and Chronic Pelvic Pain Syndrome

1. "Prostatitis: Inflammation of the Prostate," NIDDK, July 2014, https://www.niddk.nih.gov/health-information/urologic-diseases/prostate-problems/prostatitis-inflammation-prostate.

2. Jonathan Bergman and Scott I. Zeitlin, "Prostatitis and Chronic Prostatitis/Chronic Pelvic Pain Syndrome," *Expert Review of Neurotherapeutics* 7, no. 3 (2007): 301–7, doi: 10.1586/14737175.7.3.301.

3. Kyung Seop Lee and Jae Duck Choi, "Chronic Prostatitis: Approaches for Best Management," *Korean Journal of Urology* 53, no. 2 (2012): 69–77, doi: 10.4111/kju.2012.53.2.69.

4. Timothy J. Coker and Daniel D. Dierfeldt, "Acute Bacterial Prostatitis: Diagnosis and Management," *American Family Physician* 93, no. 2 (2016): 114–20.

5. Samuel G. Deem et al., "Acute Bacterial Prostatitis Clinical Presentation: History, Physical," Medscape, September 7, 2018, https://emedicine.medscape.com/article/2002872-clinical.

6. Coker and Dierfeldt, "Acute Bacterial Prostatitis"; and Paul J. Turek, Tarlan Hedayati, and Christine R. Stehman, "Prostatitis Clinical Presentation: History, Physical Examination, Complications," Medscape, November 1, 2019, https://emedicine.medscape.com /article/785418-clinical.

7. Turek, Hedayati, and Stehman, "Prostatitis Clinical Presentation."

8. Coker and Dierfeldt, "Acute Bacterial Prostatitis."

9. Deem et al., "Acute Bacterial Prostatitis Clinical Presentation."

10. Noel L. Smith et al., "Ozone Therapy: An Overview of Pharmacodynamics, Current Research, and Clinical Utility," *Medical Gas Research* 7, no. 3 (2017): 212–19, doi: 10.4103/2045-9912.215752.

11. James D. Holt et al., "Common Questions about Chronic Prostatitis," *American Family Physician* 93, no. 4 (2016): 290–96.

12. Samantha D. Kraemer and Sugandh Shetty, "Chronic Bacterial Prostatitis: Practice Essentials, Background, Anatomy and Physiology," Medscape, January 15, 2019, https://emedicine .medscape.com/article/458391-overview.

13. Kraemer and Shetty, "Chronic Bacterial Prostatitis."

14. Kraemer and Shetty, "Chronic Bacterial Prostatitis."

15. Kraemer and Shetty, "Chronic Bacterial Prostatitis."

16. Holt et al., "Common Questions."

17. Paul S. Anderson, "Biofilms: What Have We Learned from the Research?" Naturopathic Doctor News and Review, January 2, 2018, https://ndnr.com/gastrointestinal /biofilms-what-have-we-learned-from-the-research.

18. Jon Rees et al., "Diagnosis and Treatment of Chronic Bacterial Prostatitis and Chronic Prostatitis/Chronic Pelvic Pain Syndrome: A Consensus Guideline," *BJU International* 116, no. 4 (2015): 509–25, doi: 10.1111/bju.13101.

19. Tommaso Cai et al., "*Serenoa repens* Associated with *Urtica dioica* (Prostamev®) and Curcumin and Quercitin (Flogmev®) Extracts Are Able to Improve the Efficacy of Prulifloxacin in Bacterial Prostatitis Patients: Results from a Prospective Randomised Study,"

International Journal of Antimicrobial Agents 33, no. 6 (2009): 549–53, doi: 10.1016/j.ijantimicag.2008.11.012.

20. Richard A. Watson, "Chronic Pelvic Pain in Men: Practice Essentials, Etiology, Epidemiology," Medscape, March 17, 2020, https://emedicine.medscape.com/article/437745-overview.

21. Watson, "Chronic Pelvic Pain."

22. Watson, "Chronic Pelvic Pain."

23. Holt et al., "Common Questions."

24. Yadong Zhang et al., "Erectile Dysfunction in Chronic Prostatitis/Chronic Pelvic Pain Syndrome: Outcomes from a Multi-Center Study and Risk Factor Analysis in a Single Center," *PLOS ONE* 11, no. 4 (2016): e0153054, doi: 10.1371/journal.pone.0153054.

25. "A Guide to the Pelvic Floor Muscles—Men," Oxford University Hospitals NHS Trust, November 2017, https://www.ouh.nhs.uk/information.

26. Riccardo Bartoletti et al., "Prevalence, Incidence Estimation, Risk Factors and Characterization of Chronic Prostatitis/Chronic Pelvic Pain Syndrome in Urological Hospital Outpatients in Italy: Results of a Multicenter Case-Control Observational Study," *Journal of Urology* 178, no. 6 (2007): 2411–15, doi: 10.1016/j.juro.2007.08.046.

27. Kyung Seop Lee and Jae Duck Choi, "Chronic Prostatitis: Approaches for Best Management," *Korean Journal of Urology* 53, no. 2 (2012): 69–77, doi: 10.4111/kju.2012.53.2.69.

28. Lee and Choi, "Chronic Prostatitis."

29. Ahmed Fouad Kotb et al., "Chronic Prostatitis/Chronic Pelvic Pain Syndrome: The Role of an Antifungal Regimen," *Central European Journal of Urology* 66, no. 2 (2013): 196–99, doi: 10.5173/ceju.2013.02.art21.

30. Sunil K. Ahuja, "Nonbacterial Prostatitis Medication," Medscape, November 25, 2019, https://emedicine.medscape.com/article/456165-medication.

31. R. Christopher Doiron and J. Curtis Nickel, "Management of Chronic Prostatitis/Chronic Pelvic Pain Syndrome," *Canadian Urological Association Journal* 12, no. 6S3 (2018): S161–63, doi: 10.5489/cuaj.5325.

32. "Prostatitis (Infection of the Prostate): Symptoms, Diagnosis & Treatment," Urology Care Foundation, https://www.urologyhealth.org/urologic-conditions/prostatitis-(infection-of-the-prostate).

33. "Yeast Infection," Johns Hopkins Medicine, https://www
.hopkinsmedicine.org/health/conditions-and-diseases/candidiasis
-yeast-infection.

34. Qiangdong Guan et al., "The Effect of Flavonoids on Chronic
Prostatitis: A Meta-Analysis of Published Randomized Controlled
Trials," *Journal of the National Medical Association* 111, no. 5 (2019):
555–62, doi: 10.1016/j.jnma.2019.04.007.

35. Florian M. E. Wagenlehner et al., "Pollen Extract for Chronic
Prostatitis—Chronic Pelvic Pain Syndrome," *Urologic Clinics
of North America* 38, no. 3 (2011): 285–92, doi: 10.1016
/j.ucl.2011.04.004.

36. Tommaso Cai et al., "The Role of Flower Pollen Extract in
Managing Patients Affected by Chronic Prostatitis/Chronic
Pelvic Pain Syndrome: A Comprehensive Analysis of All
Published Clinical Trials," *BMC Urology* 17, no. 1 (2017),
doi: 10.1186/s12894-017-0223-5.

37. Cai et al., "Role of Flower Pollen Extract."

38. E. W. Rugendorff et al., "Results of Treatment with Pollen
Extract (Cernilton N) in Chronic Prostatitis and Prostatodynia,"
British Journal of Urology 71, no. 4 (1993): 433–38, doi:
10.1111/j.1464-410x.1993.tb15988x.

39. G. Morgia et al., "Treatment of Chronic Prostatitis/Chronic Pelvic
Pain Syndrome Category IIIA with *Serenoa repens* plus Selenium and
Lycopene (Profluss®) versus *S. repens* Alone: An Italian Randomized
Multicenter-Controlled Study," *Urologia Internationalis* 84, no. 4
(2010): 400–406, doi: 10.1159/000302716.

40. Nicola Macchione et al., "Flower Pollen Extract in Association
with Vitamins (Deprox 500®) versus *Serenoa repens* in Chronic
Prostatitis/Chronic Pelvic Pain Syndrome: A Comparative Analysis
of Two Different Treatments," *Anti-Inflammatory & Anti-Allergy
Agents in Medicinal Chemistry* 18, no. 2 (2019): 151–61, doi: 10.2174
/1871523018666181128164252.

41. Jane Higdon et al., "Flavonoids," Linus Pauling Institute,
February 2016, https://lpi.oregonstate.edu/mic/dietary
-factors/phytochemicals/flavonoids.

42. Gianni Paulis, "Inflammatory Mechanisms and Oxidative Stress in
Prostatitis: The Possible Role of Antioxidant Therapy," *Research and
Reports in Urology* 10 (2018): 75–87, doi: 10.2147/rru.s170400.

43. Daniel A. Shoskes et al., "Quercetin in Men with Category III
Chronic Prostatitis: A Preliminary Prospective, Double-Blind,
Placebo-Controlled Trial," *Urology* 54, no. 6 (1999): 960–63,
doi: 10.1016/s0090-4295(99)00358-1.

44. Angela Maurizi et al., "The Role of Nutraceutical Medications in Men with Non Bacterial Chronic Prostatitis and Chronic Pelvic Pain Syndrome: A Prospective Non Blinded Study Utilizing Flower Pollen Extracts versus Bioflavonoids," *Archivio Italiano di Urologia e Andrologia* 90, no. 4 (2018): 260–64, doi: 10.4081/aiua.2018.4.260.

45. Hong Li, Andrew Hung, and Angela Wei Hong Yang, "A Classic Herbal Formula Danggui Beimu Kushen Wan for Chronic Prostatitis: From Traditional Knowledge to Scientific Exploration," *Evidence-Based Complementary and Alternative Medicine* 2018 (2018): 1–11, doi: 10.1155/2018/1612948.

46. Amin S. Herati et al., "Effects of Foods and Beverages on the Symptoms of Chronic Prostatitis/Chronic Pelvic Pain Syndrome," *Urology* 82, no. 6 (2013): 1376–80, doi: 10.1016 /j.urology.2013.07.015.

47. Zongshi Qin et al., "Acupuncture for Chronic Prostatitis/Chronic Pelvic Pain Syndrome: A Randomized, Sham Acupuncture Controlled Trial," *Journal of Urology* 200, no. 4 (2018): 815–22, doi: 10.1016/j.juro.2018.05.001.

48. Rodney U. Anderson et al., "Integration of Myofascial Trigger Point Release and Paradoxical Relaxation Training Treatment of Chronic Pelvic Pain in Men," *Journal of Urology* 174, no. 1 (2005): 155–60, doi: 10.1097/01.ju.0000161609.31185.d5.

49. "OMT: Osteopathic Manipulative Treatment | American Osteopathic Association," American Osteopathic Association, https://osteopathic.org/what-is-osteopathic-medicine/osteopathic -manipulative-treatment.

50. Sylvia Marx, "Does Osteopathic Treatment Have an Influence on the Symptoms of Patients with Chronic Prostatitis/Chronic Pelvic Pain Syndrome (CPPS)? A Randomized Controlled Trial," *International Journal of Osteopathic Medicine* 9, no. 1 (2006): 44, doi: 10.1016/j.ijosm.2006.01.022.

51. Paul J. Turek, Tarlan Hedayati, and Christine R. Stehman, "How Is Asymptomatic Inflammatory Prostatitis Characterized?" Medscape, November 1, 2019, https://www.medscape.com /answers/785418-60712/how-is-asymptomatic-inflammatory -prostatitis-characterized.

52. Rikiya Taoka and Yoshiyuki Kakehi, "The Influence of Asymptomatic Inflammatory Prostatitis on the Onset and Progression of Lower Urinary Tract Symptoms in Men with Histologic Benign Prostatic Hyperplasia," *Asian Journal of Urology* 4, no. 3 (2017): 158–63, doi: 10.1016/j.ajur.2017.02.004.

53. Taoka and Kakehi, "The Influence of Asymptomatic Inflammatory Prostatitis."

54. Taoka and Kakehi, "The Influence of Asymptomatic Inflammatory Prostatitis."

Chapter 5: Prostate Cancer

1. "Key Statistics for Prostate Cancer," Cancer.org, January 8, 2020, https://www.cancer.org/cancer/prostate-cancer/about/key-statistics .html.

2. James L. Mohler et al., "Prostate Cancer, Version 2.2019, NCCN Clinical Practice Guidelines in Oncology," *Journal of the National Comprehensive Cancer Network* 17, no. 5 (2019): 479–505, doi: 10.6004/jnccn.2019.0023.

3. "Key Statistics for Prostate Cancer," Cancer.org.

4. "Prostate Cancer: Risk Factors and Prevention," Cancer.net, American Society of Clinical Oncology, November 2019, https:// www.cancer.net/cancer-types/prostate-cancer/risk-factors -and-prevention; and "Prostate Cancer Risk Factors," Prostate Cancer Foundation, https://www.pcf.org/patient-resources /family-cancer-risk/prostate-cancer-risk-factors.

5. Mohler et al., "Prostate Cancer, Version 2.2019."

6. "Tests to Diagnose and Stage Prostate Cancer," American Cancer Society, January 30, 2020, https://www.cancer.org/cancer/prostate -cancer/detection-diagnosis-staging/how-diagnosed.html.

7. "Tests to Diagnose," American Cancer Society.

8. Eric J. Topol and Richard J. Ablin, "PSA Test Is Misused, Unreliable, Says the Antigen's Discoverer," Medscape, August 8, 2014, https:// www.medscape.com/viewarticle/828854_4.

9. Mohler et al., "Prostate Cancer, Version 2.2019."

10. "Prostate-Specific Antigen (PSA) Test," National Cancer Institute at the National Institutes of Health, October 4, 2017, https://www .cancer.gov/types/prostate/psa-fact-sheet.

11. Richard M. Martin et al., "Effect of a Low-Intensity PSA-Based Screening Intervention on Prostate Cancer Mortality," *JAMA* 319, no. 9 (2018): 883–95, doi: 10.1001/jama.2018.0154.

12. Kirsten Bibbins-Domingo, David C. Grossman, and Susan J. Curry, "The US Preventive Services Task Force 2017 Draft

Recommendation Statement on Screening for Prostate Cancer,"
JAMA 317, no. 19 (2017): 1949–50, doi: 10.1001/jama.2017.4413.

13. "Screening Tests for Prostate Cancer," American Cancer Society,
August 1, 2019, https://www.cancer.org/cancer/prostate-cancer
/detection-diagnosis-staging/tests.html.

14. "Screening Tests for Prostate Cancer," American Cancer Society.

15. "Screening Tests for Prostate Cancer," American Cancer Society.

16. "Screening Tests for Prostate Cancer," American Cancer Society.

17. "Prostate-Specific Antigen (PSA) Test," National Cancer Institute.

18. "Understanding Your Pathology Report: Prostate Cancer,"
American Cancer Society, March 8, 2017, https://www.cancer.org
/treatment/understanding-your-diagnosis/tests/understanding
-your-pathology-report/prostate-pathology/prostate-cancer
-pathology.html.

19. "Understanding Your Pathology Report," American Cancer Society.

20. "Understanding Your Pathology Report," American Cancer Society.

21. "Understanding Your Pathology Report," American Cancer Society.

22. "Understanding Your Pathology Report," American Cancer Society.

23. "Understanding Your Pathology Report," American Cancer Society;
and "Prostate Cancer: Diagnosis," Cancer.net, American Society of
Clinical Oncology, November 2019, https://www.cancer.net
/cancer-types/prostate-cancer/diagnosis.

24. "Prostate Cancer: Types of Treatment," Cancer.net, American
Society of Clinical Oncology, November 2019, https://www.cancer
.net/cancer-types/prostate-cancer/types-treatment.

25. "Treating Prostate Cancer," American Cancer Society, https://www
.cancer.org/cancer/prostate-cancer/treating.html.

26. "Active Surveillance," Prostate Cancer Foundation, https://www.
pcf.org/about-prostate-cancer/prostate-cancer-treatment
/active-surveillance.

27. "Treating Prostate Cancer," American Cancer Society, https://www
.cancer.org/cancer/prostate-cancer/treating.html.

28. National Cancer Institute, "Prostate Cancer, Nutrition, and Dietary
Supplements (PDQ®): Integrative, Alternative, and Complementary
Therapies - Patient Information [NCI]," UW Health, November
2019, https://www.uwhealth.org/health/topic/nci/prostate
-cancer-nutrition-and-dietary-supplements-pdq-integrative

-alternative-and-complementary-therapies-patient-information
-nci/ncicdr0000719565.html.

29. Donald I. Abrams, "An Integrative Approach to Prostate Cancer," *Journal of Alternative and Complementary Medicine* 24, nos. 9–10 (2018): 872–80, doi: 10.1089/acm.2018.0169.

30. Mark Stengler and Paul Anderson, *Outside the Box Cancer Therapies* (Carlsbad: Hay House, 2018).

31. "Cancer Causes and Prevention, Risk Factors: Chronic Inflammation," National Cancer Institute at the National Institutes of Health, April 29, 2015, https://www.cancer.gov/about-cancer /causes-prevention/risk/chronic-inflammation.

32. Dean Ornish et al., "Intensive Lifestyle Changes May Affect the Progression of Prostate Cancer," *Journal of Urology* 174, no. 3 (2005): 1065–70, doi: 10.1097/01.ju.0000169487.49018.73.

33. Ornish et al., "Intensive Lifestyle Changes."

34. Justin R. Gregg et al., "Diet Quality and Gleason Grade Progression among Localised Prostate Cancer Patients on Active Surveillance," *British Journal of Cancer* 120, no. 4 (2019): 466–71, doi: 10.1038 /s41416-019-0380-2.

35. Stacey A. Kenfield et al., "Mediterranean Diet and Prostate Cancer Risk and Mortality in the Health Professionals Follow-Up Study," *European Urology* 65, no. 5 (2014): 887–94, doi: 10.1016 /j.eururo.2013.08.009.

36. Kenfield et al., "Mediterranean Diet and Prostate Cancer Risk."

37. Kenfield et al., "Mediterranean Diet and Prostate Cancer Risk."

38. Giorgio Ivan Russo et al., "Adherence to Mediterranean Diet and Prostate Cancer Risk in Sicily: Population-Based Case–Control Study," *International Journal of Impotence Research* 31, no. 4 (2018): 269–75, doi: 10.1038/s41443-018-0088-5.

39. Adela Castelló et al., "Mediterranean Dietary Pattern Is Associated with Low Risk of Aggressive Prostate Cancer: MCC-Spain Study," *Journal of Urology* 199, no. 2 (2018): 430–37, doi: 10.1016/j.juro.2017.08.087.

40. Castelló et al., "Mediterranean Dietary Pattern."

41. Russo et al., "Adherence to Mediterranean Diet."

42. Yuming Guo et al., "Green Tea and the Risk of Prostate Cancer," *Medicine* 96, no. 13 (2017): e6426, doi: 10.1097 /md.0000000000006426.

43. Maurizio Muscaritoli et al., "Prevalence of Malnutrition in Patients at First Medical Oncology Visit: The PreMiO Study," *Oncotarget* 8, no. 45 (2017), doi: 10.18632/oncotarget.20168.

44. Donald L. Trump and Jeanny B. Aragon-Ching, "Vitamin D in Prostate Cancer," *Asian Journal of Andrology* 20, no. 3 (2018): 244–52, doi: 10.4103/aja.aja_14_18.

45. Trump and Aragon-Ching, "Vitamin D in Prostate Cancer."

46. Zhen-yu Song et al., "Circulating Vitamin D Level and Mortality in Prostate Cancer Patients: A Dose-Response Meta-Analysis," *Endocrine Connections* 7, no. 12 (2018): R294–303, doi: 10.1530/ec-18-0283.

47. K. W. Tsang et al., "*Coriolus versicolor* Polysaccharide Peptide Slows Progression of Advanced Non-Small Cell Lung Cancer," *Respiratory Medicine* 97, no. 6 (2003): 618–24, doi: 10.1053/rmed.2003.1490.

48. Jennifer Man-Fan Wan et al., "Polysaccharopeptides Derived from *Coriolus versicolor* Potentiate the S-Phase Specific Cytotoxicity of Camptothecin (CPT) on Human Leukemia HL-60 Cells," *Chinese Medicine* 5, no. 1 (2010): 16, doi: 10.1186/1749-8546-5-16.

49. Parris M. Kidd, "The Use of Mushroom Glucans and Proteoglycans in Cancer Treatment," *Alternative Medicine Review* 5, no. 1 (2000): 4–27.

50. Z. Sun et al., "The Ameliorative Effect of PSP on the Toxic and Side Reaction of Chemo- and Radiotherapy of Cancers," in *Advanced Research in PSP*, ed. Q. Yang (Hong Kong: Hong Kong Association for Health Care, 1999).

51. Mark Mayell, "Maitake Extracts and Their Therapeutic Potential: A Review," *Alternative Medicine Review* 6, no. 1 (2001): 51; Masuda et al., "Inhibitory Effect of MD-Fraction on Tumor Metastasis: Involvement of NK Cell Activation and Suppression of Intercellular Adhesion Molecule (ICAM)-1 Expression in Lung Vascular Endothelial Cells," *Biological and Pharmaceutical Bulletin* 31, no. 6 (2008):1104–8, doi: 10.1248/bpb.31.1104; and "Maitake," Memorial Sloan Kettering Cancer Center, February 19, 2020, https://www.mskcc.org/cancer-care/integrative-medicine/herbs/maitake.

52. Hiroaki Nanba, *Maitake Challenges Cancer* (Kobe, Japan: Socio Health Group, 1998).

53. Vladislav V. Glinsky and Avraham Raz, "Modified Citrus Pectin Anti-Metastatic Properties: One Bullet, Multiple Targets," *Carbohydrate Research* 344, no. 14 (2009): 1788–91, doi: 10.1016/j.carres.2008.08.038.

54. Pratima Nangia-Makker et al., "Galectin-3 Binding and Metastasis," *Methods in Molecular Biology* 878 (2012): 251–66, doi: 10.1007/978-1-61779-854-2_17.

55. Cheppail Ramachandran et al., "Activation of Human T-Helper/ Inducer Cell, T-Cytotoxic Cell, B-cell, and Natural Killer (NK)- Cells and Induction of Natural Killer Cell Activity against K562 Chronic Myeloid Leukemia Cells with Modified Citrus Pectin," *BMC Complementary and Alternative Medicine* 11 (2011), doi: 10.1186/1472-6882-11-59.

56. B. W. Guess et al., "Modified Citrus Pectin (MCP) Increases the Prostate-Specific Antigen Doubling Time in Men with Prostate Cancer: A Phase II Pilot Study," *Prostate Cancer and Prostatic Diseases* 6, no. 4 (2003): 301–4, doi: 10.1038/sj.pcan.4500679.

57. Jun Yan and Aaron Katz, "PectaSol-C Modified Citrus Pectin Induces Apoptosis and Inhibition of Proliferation in Human and Mouse Androgen-Dependent and Independent Prostate Cancer Cells," *Integrative Cancer Therapies* 9, no. 2 (2010): 197–203, doi: 10.1177/1534735410369672.

58. Jung-Mi Yun, Ishwarlal Jialal, and Sridevi Devaraj, "Epigenetic Regulation of High Glucose-Induced Proinflammatory Cytokine Production in Monocytes by Curcumin," *The Journal of Nutritional Biochemistry* 22, no. 5 (2011): 450–58, doi: 10.1016 /j.jnutbio.2010.03.014.

59. Jane Higdon et al., "Curcumin," Linus Pauling Institute, March 2016, http://lpi.oregonstate.edu/mic/dietary-factors /phytochemicals/curcumin.

60. Karthik Gridhar, "Curcumin: Can It Slow Cancer Growth?" Mayo Clinic, March 11, 2020, https://www.mayoclinic.org /diseases-conditions/cancer/expert-answers/curcumin /faq-20057858.

61. Walter Lemmo and Gerard Tan, "Prolonged Survival after Dichloroacetate Treatment of Non-Small-Cell Lung Carcinoma- Related Leptomeningeal Carcinomatosis," *Journal of Medical Cases* 7, no. 4 (2016): 136–42, doi: 10.14740/jmc2456w.

62. Akbar Khan, "Case Report of Long Term Complete Remission of Metastatic Renal Squamous Cell Carcinoma after Palliative Radiotherapy and Adjuvant Dichloroacetate," *Advances in Cancer Research & Treatment*, (2013), doi: 10.5171/2012.441895.

63. NCI Staff, "Prescribing Exercise as Cancer Treatment: A Conversation with Dr. Kathryn Schmitz," National Cancer Institute at the National Institutes of Health, November 12, 2019, https://www.cancer.gov/news-events/cancer-currents-blog /2019/cancer-survivors-exercise-guidelines-schmitz.

64. NCI Staff, "Prescribing Exercise as Cancer Treatment."

65. NCI Staff, "Prescribing Exercise as Cancer Treatment."

66. Michael Hiroshi Johnson, "Combat Prostate Cancer with Exercise," Johns Hopkins Medicine, https://www.hopkinsmedicine.org /health/conditions-and-diseases/prostate-cancer/combat -prostate-cancer-with-exercise.

67. Stacey A. Kenfield et al., "Physical Activity and Survival after Prostate Cancer Diagnosis in the Health Professionals Follow-Up Study," *Journal of Clinical Oncology* 29, no. 6 (2011): 726–32, doi: 10.1200/jco.2010.31.5226.

68. Yoichi Chida et al., "Do Stress-Related Psychosocial Factors Contribute to Cancer Incidence and Survival?" *Nature Clinical Practice Oncology* 5, no. 8 (2008): 466–75, doi: 10.1038/ncponc1134.

69. Qi Chen et al., "Pharmacologic Ascorbic Acid Concentrations Selectively Kill Cancer Cells: Action as a Pro-Drug to Deliver Hydrogen Peroxide to Tissues," *Proceedings of the National Academy of Sciences* 102, no. 38 (2005): 13604–9, doi: 10.1073/pnas.0506390102.

70. Ron Hunninghake, "Adjunctive IVC Therapy Help Cancer Patients Update," 3rd Annual Conference and Expo IV Therapies 2014 Integrative Oncology, January 25, 2014; and Nina A. Mikirova et al., "Intravenous Ascorbic Acid Protocol for Cancer Patients: Scientific Rationale, Pharmacology, and Clinical Experience," *Functional Foods in Health and Disease* 3, no. 8 (2013): 344–66, doi: 10.31989/ffhd.v3i8.43.

71. Anitra C. Carr, Margreet C. M. Vissers, and John S. Cook, "The Effect of Intravenous Vitamin C on Cancer- and Chemotherapy-Related Fatigue and Quality of Life," *Frontiers in Oncology* 4 (2014), doi: 10.3389/fonc.2014.00283.

Chapter 6: The Testosterone Factor

1. "Low Testosterone (Male Hypogonadism): Causes, Symptoms, Diagnosis & Treatment," Cleveland Clinic, reviewed April 10, 2018, https://my.clevelandclinic.org/health/diseases /15603-low-testosterone-male-hypogonadism.

2. "What is Erectile Dysfunction?," Urology Care Foundation, updated June 2018, https://www.urologyhealth.org/urologic -conditions/erectile-dysfunction.

3. Gail A. Laughlin, Elizabeth Barrett-Connor, and Jaclyn Bergstrom, "Low Serum Testosterone and Mortality in Older Men," *The Journal*

of Clinical Endocrinology & Metabolism 93, no. 1 (2008): 68–75, doi: 10.1210/jc.2007-1792.

4. Matthew Solan, "Treating Low Testosterone Levels," Harvard Health Publishing, updated August 9, 2019, https://www.health .harvard.edu/mens-health/treating-low-testosterone-levels.

5. "Male 'Menopause,'" WebMD, reviewed February 11, 2019, https:// www.webmd.com/men/guide/male-menopause.

6. Parminder Singh, "Andropause: Current Concepts," *Indian Journal of Endocrinology and Metabolism* 17, no. 9 (2013): 621–29, doi: 10.4103/2230-8210.123552.

7. Maria G. Vogiatzi, "Hypogonadism: Practice Essentials, Background, Pathophysiology," Medscape, updated April 3, 2019, https://emedicine.medscape.com/article/922038-overview.

8. Schlomo Melmed et al., *Williams Textbook of Endocrinology*, 13th ed. reprint (Philadelphia, PA: Elsevier, 2016).

9. Andre B. Araujo et al., "Endogenous Testosterone and Mortality in Men: A Systematic Review and Meta-Analysis," *The Journal of Clinical Endocrinology & Metabolism* 96, no. 10 (2011): 3007–19, doi: 10.1210/jc.2011-1137.

10. Laughlin, Barrett-Connor, and Bergstrom, "Low Serum Testosterone and Mortality."

11. Molly M. Shores et al., "Low Serum Testosterone and Mortality in Male Veterans," *Archives of Internal Medicine* 166, no. 15 (2006): 1660–65, doi: 10.1001/archinte.166.15.1660.

12. Kay-Tee Khaw et al., "Endogenous Testosterone and Mortality Due to All Causes, Cardiovascular Disease, and Cancer in Men," *Circulation* 116, no. 23 (2007): 2694–701, doi: 10.1161 /circulationaha.107.719005.

13. Vakkat Muraleedharan et al., "Testosterone Deficiency Is Associated with Increased Risk of Mortality and Testosterone Replacement Improves Survival in Men with Type 2 Diabetes," *European Journal of Endocrinology* 169, no. 6 (2013): 725–33, doi: 10.1530/eje-13-0321.

14. Richard Casaburi et al., "Effects of Testosterone and Resistance Training in Men with Chronic Obstructive Pulmonary Disease," *American Journal of Respiratory and Critical Care Medicine* 170, no. 8 (2004): 870–78, doi: 10.1164/rccm.200305-617oc; and Ian R. Reid, "Testosterone Therapy in Glucocorticoid-Treated Men," *Archives of Internal Medicine* 156, no. 11 (1996): 1173–77, doi: 10.1001 /archinte.1996.00440100065008.

15. John Kyriazis et al., "Low Serum Testosterone, Arterial Stiffness and Mortality in Male Haemodialysis Patients," *Nephrology Dialysis Transplantation* 26, no. 9 (2011): 2971–77, doi: 10.1093/ndt/gfq847.

16. John P. Mulhall et al., "Evaluation and Management of Testosterone Deficiency: AUA Guideline," *Journal of Urology* 200, no. 2 (2018): 423–32, doi: 10.1016/j.juro.2018.03.115; and Shalender Bhasin et al., "Testosterone Therapy in Men with Hypogonadism: An Endocrine Society Clinical Practice Guideline," *The Journal of Clinical Endocrinology & Metabolism* 103, no. 5 (2018): 1715–44, doi: 10.1210/jc.2018-00229.

17. Mulhall et al., "Evaluation and Management."

18. Mulhall et al., "Evaluation and Management."

19. Bhasin et al., "Testosterone Therapy."

20. Vineet Tyagi et al., "Revisiting the Role of Testosterone: Are We Missing Something?," *Reviews in Urology* 19, no. 1 (2017): 16–24, doi: 10.3909/riu0716.

21. Tyagi et al., "Revisiting the Role of Testosterone."

22. Tyagi et al., "Revisiting the Role of Testosterone."

23. Melmed et al., *Williams Textbook of Endocrinology.*

24. Melmed et al., *Williams Textbook of Endocrinology.*

25. Melmed et al., *Williams Textbook of Endocrinology.*

26. Vogiatzi, "Hypogonadism."

27. Bhasin et al., "Testosterone Therapy"; and Saba Rehman et al., "Endocrine Disrupting Chemicals and Impact on Male Reproductive Health," *Translational Andrology and Urology* 7, no. 3 (2018): 490–503, doi: 10.21037/tau.2018.05.17.

28. "Can Prescription Medications Affect Testosterone Levels?" International Society for Sexual Medicine, https://www.issm .info/sexual-health-qa/can-prescription-medications-affect -testosterone-levels.

29. Bhasin et al., "Testosterone Therapy."

30. Rehman et al., "Endocrine Disrupting Chemicals."

31. Rehman et al., "Endocrine Disrupting Chemicals."

32. Rehman et al., "Endocrine Disrupting Chemicals."

33. Rehman et al., "Endocrine Disrupting Chemicals."

34. Rehman et al., "Endocrine Disrupting Chemicals."

35. Rehman et al., "Endocrine Disrupting Chemicals."

36. Rehman et al., "Endocrine Disrupting Chemicals."

37. John D. Meeker et al., "Exposure to Nonpersistent Insecticides and Male Reproductive Hormones," *Epidemiology* 17, no. 1 (2006): 61–68, doi: 10.1097/01.ede.0000190602.14691.70.

38. Priyanka Roy et al., "Pesticides, Insecticides and Male Infertility," *International Journal of Reproduction, Contraception, Obstetrics and Gynecology* 6, no. 8 (2017): 3387, doi: 10.18203/2320 -1770.ijrcog20173448.

39. Kevin M. Rice et al., "Environmental Mercury and Its Toxic Effects," *Journal of Preventive Medicine & Public Health* 47, no. 2 (2014): 74–83, doi: 10.3961/jpmph.2014.47.2.74.

40. Mohit Khera et al., "Diagnosis and Treatment of Testosterone Deficiency: Recommendations from The Fourth International Consultation for Sexual Medicine (ICSM 2015)," *The Journal of Sexual Medicine* 13, no. 12 (2016): 1787–1804, doi: 10.1016 /j.jsxm.2016.10.009.

41. Mulhall et al., "Evaluation and Management"; and Bhasin et al., "Testosterone Therapy."

42. Bhasin et al., "Testosterone Therapy."

43. Bhasin et al., "Testosterone Therapy."

44. "Just for Men," National Osteoporosis Foundation, https://www .nof.org/preventing-fractures/general-facts/just-for-men.

45. Tzu-Yu Hu et al., "Testosterone-Associated Dietary Pattern Predicts Low Testosterone Levels and Hypogonadism," *Nutrients* 10, no. 11 (2018): 1786, doi: 10.3390/nu10111786.

46. Hu et al., "Testosterone-Associated Dietary Pattern."

47. Premal Patel et al., "Impaired Sleep Is Associated with Low Testosterone in US Adult Males: Results from the National Health and Nutrition Examination Survey," *World Journal of Urology* 37, no. 7 (2018): 1449–53, doi: 10.1007/s00345-018-2485-2.

48. Jeong Kyun Yeo et al., "Which Exercise Is Better for Increasing Serum Testosterone Levels in Patients with Erectile Dysfunction?" *The World Journal of Men's Health* 36, no. 2 (2018): 147–52, doi: 10.5534/wjmh.17030.

49. Dae-Yeon Cho et al., "Exercise Improves the Effects of Testosterone Replacement Therapy and the Durability of Response after Cessation of Treatment: A Pilot Randomized Controlled Trial," *Asian Journal of Andrology* 19, no. 5 (2017): 602–07, doi: 10.4103/1008-682x.184269.

50. Sachin Wankhede et al., "Examining the Effect of *Withania somnifera* Supplementation on Muscle Strength and Recovery: A Randomized Controlled Trial," *Journal of the International Society of Sports Nutrition* 12, no. 43 (2015), doi: 10.1186/s12970-015-0104-9.

51. Lakshmi-Chandra Mishra, Betsy B. Singh, and Simon Dagenais, "Scientific Basis for the Therapeutic Use of *Withania somnifera* (Ashwagandha): A Review," *Alternative Medicine Review* 5, no. 4 (2000): 334–46.

52. Biswajit Auddy et al., "A Standardized *Withania somnifera* Extract Significantly Reduces Stress-Related Parameters in Chronically Stressed Humans: A Double-Blind, Randomized, Placebo-Controlled Study," *Journal of the American Nutraceutical Association* 11, no. 1 (2008): 51–57.

53. Vijay R. Ambiye et al., "Clinical Evaluation of the Spermatogenic Activity of the Root Extract of Ashwagandha (*Withania somnifera*) in Oligospermic Males: A Pilot Study," *Evidence-Based Complementary and Alternative Medicine*, (2013), 1–6, doi: 10.1155/2013/571420.

54. Wankhede et al., "Effect of *Withania somnifera* Supplementation."

55. Committee on Herbal Medicinal Products (HMPC), "Reflection Paper on the Adaptogenic Concept," European Medicines Agency, 2008, https://www.ema.europa.eu/en/documents/scientific -guideline/reflection-paper-adaptogenic-concept_en.pdf.

56. Wankhede et al., "Effect of *Withania somnifera* Supplementation"; and Auddy et al., "Standardized *Withania somnifera* Extract."

57. Wankhede et al., "Effect of *Withania somnifera* Supplementation."

58. Wankhede et al., "Effect of *Withania somnifera* Supplementation."

59. Ambiye et al., "Spermatogenic Activity."

60. Adrian L. Lopresti, Peter D. Drummond, and Stephen J. Smith, "A Randomized, Double-Blind, Placebo-Controlled, Crossover Study Examining the Hormonal and Vitality Effects of Ashwagandha (*Withania somnifera*) in Aging, Overweight Males," *American Journal of Men's Health* 13, no. 2 (2019): 155798831983598, doi: 10.1177/1557988319835985.

61. Shawn M. Talbott et al., "Effect of Tongkat Ali on Stress Hormones and Psychological Mood State in Moderately Stressed Subjects," *Journal of the International Society of Sports Nutrition* 10, no. 1 (2013): 28, doi: 10.1186/1550-2783-10-28.

62. Hnin Ei Thu et al., "*Eurycoma longifolia* as a Potential Adoptogen of Male Sexual Health: A Systematic Review on Clinical Studies,"

Chinese Journal of Natural Medicines 15, no. 1 (2017): 71–80, doi: 10.1016/s1875-5364(17)30010-9.

63. Talbott et al., "Effect of Tongkat Ali"; and Ralf R. Henkel et al., "Tongkat Ali as a Potential Herbal Supplement for Physically Active Male and Female Seniors—a Pilot Study," *Phytotherapy Research* 28, no. 4 (2013): 544–50, doi: 10.1002/ptr.5017.

64. Talbott et al., "Effect of Tongkat Ali."

65. Henkel et al., "Tongkat Ali as a Potential Herbal Supplement."

66. Talbott et al., "Effect of Tongkat Ali."

67. Thu et al., "*Eurycoma longifolia* as a Potential Adoptogen."

68. Michael T. Murray and Joseph E. Pizzorno, *The Encyclopedia of Natural Medicine*, reprint (New York: Atria Books, 2012).

69. Ananda S. Prasad et al., "Zinc Status and Serum Testosterone Levels of Healthy Adults," *Nutrition* 12, no. 5 (1996): 344–48, doi: 10.1016/s0899-9007(96)80058-x.

70. Vedat Cinar et al., "Effects of Magnesium Supplementation on Testosterone Levels of Athletes and Sedentary Subjects at Rest and after Exhaustion," *Biological Trace Element Research* 140, no. 1 (2010): 18–23, doi: 10.1007/s12011-010-8676-3.

71. Mulhall et al., "Evaluation and Management"; and Bhasin et al., "Testosterone Therapy."

72. Bhasin et al., "Testosterone Therapy."

73. Bhasin et al., "Testosterone Therapy."

74. Hyun Jun Park, Sun Tae Ahn, and Du Geon Moon, "Evolution of Guidelines for Testosterone Replacement Therapy," *Journal of Clinical Medicine* 8, no. 3 (2019): 410, doi: 10.3390/jcm8030410.

75. Andrew W. Roddam, "Endogenous Sex Hormones and Prostate Cancer: A Collaborative Analysis of 18 Prospective Studies," *JNCI: Journal of the National Cancer Institute* 100, no. 3 (2008): 170–83, doi: 10.1093/jnci/djm323.

76. Alexander W. Pastuszak et al., "Testosterone Replacement Therapy in Patients with Prostate Cancer after Radical Prostatectomy," *Journal of Urology* 190, no. 2 (2013): 639–44, doi: 10.1016/j.juro.2013.02.002.

77. Felipe G. Balbontin et al., "Long-Acting Testosterone Injections for Treatment of Testosterone Deficiency after Brachytherapy for Prostate Cancer," *BJU International* 114, no. 1 (2014): 125–30, doi: 10.1111/bju.12668.

78. Michael A. Bell et al., "Shifting the Paradigm of Testosterone Replacement Therapy in Prostate Cancer," *The World Journal of Men's Health* 36, no. 2 (2018): 103–09, doi: 10.5534/wjmh.170007.

79. "American Association of Clinical Endocrinologists (AACE) 23rd Annual Scientific and Clinical Congress," reprint, American Association of Clinical Endocrinologists, 2014.

80. "Compounding FAQs," Alliance for Pharmacy Compounding, 2019, http://www.a4pc.org.

81. Mohamad Habous et al., "Clomiphene Citrate and Human Chorionic Gonadotropin Are Both Effective in Restoring Testosterone in Hypogonadism: A Short-Course Randomized Study," *BJU International* 122, no. 5 (2018): 889–97, doi: 10.1111/bju.14401.

Chapter 7: Erasing Erectile Dysfunction and Boosting Libido

1. Maria Yialamas and Bradley Anawalt, "Decreased Libido," Hormone.org, May 2018, https://www.hormone.org/diseases-and-conditions/decreased-libido; and "Sexual Desire Disorder," *Psychology Today*, reviewed February 7, 2019, https://www.psychologytoday.com/us/conditions/sexual-desire-disorder.

2. "Erectile Dysfunction (ED): Symptoms, Diagnosis & Treatment," Urology Care Foundation, June 2018, https://www.urologyhealth.org/urologic-conditions/erectile-dysfunction.

3. Edward David Kim and Stanley A. Brosman, "Erectile Dysfunction," Medscape, August, 8, 2018, https://emedicine.medscape.com/article/444220-overview#a5.

4. Kim and Brosman, "Erectile Dysfunction."

5. "Men with Erectile Dysfunction May Face Higher Risk of Death," Endocrine Society, March 31, 2020, https://www.endocrine.org/news-and-advocacy/news-room/2020/men-with-erectile-dysfunction-may-face-higher-risk-of-death.

6. Kim and Brosman, "Erectile Dysfunction."

7. Kim and Brosman, "Erectile Dysfunction."

8. Gholamreza Pourmand et al., "Do Cigarette Smokers with Erectile Dysfunction Benefit from Stopping?: A Prospective Study," *BJU International* 94, no. 9 (2004): 1310–13, doi: 10.1111/j.1464-410X.2004.05162.x.

9. "What Are Some Effects of Sustained Pornography Use?," International Society for Sexual Medicine, https://www.issm .info/sexual-health-qa/what-are-some-effects-of-sustained -pornography-use.

10. Berkeley Lovelace Jr., "Pfizer Still Holds the Lead in the Erectile Dysfunction Market Even as Viagra Sales Falter," CNBC, February 14, 2019, https://www.cnbc.com/2019/02/13/pfizer-holds-lead-in -erectile-dysfunction-market-as-viagra-sales-fall.html.

11. Lee Smith et al., "Participation in Physical Activity Is Associated with Sexual Activity in Older English Adults," *International Journal of Environmental Research and Public Health* 16, no. 3 (2019): 489, doi: 10.3390/ijerph16030489.

12. Simona Di Francesco and Raffaele Lanfranco Tenaglia, "Mediterranean Diet and Erectile Dysfunction: A Current Perspective," *Central European Journal of Urology* 70, no. 2 (2017): 185–87, doi: 10.5173/ceju.2017.1356.

13. K. Esposito et al., "Mediterranean Diet Improves Erectile Function in Subjects with the Metabolic Syndrome," *International Journal of Impotence Research* 18, no. 4 (2006): 405–10, doi: 10.1038/sj.ijir.3901447.

14. Arpit Koolwal et al., "L-Arginine and Erectile Dysfunction," *Journal of Psychosexual Health* 1, no. 1 (2019): 37–43, doi: 10.1177/2631831818822018.

15. Hiromitsu Aoki et al., "Clinical Assessment of a Supplement of Pycnogenol® and L-Arginine in Japanese Patients with Mild to Moderate Erectile Dysfunction," *Phytotherapy Research* 26, no. 2 (2011): 204–7, doi: 10.1002/ptr.3462; R. Stanislavov and V. Nikolova, "Treatment of Erectile Dysfunction with Pycnogenol and L-Arginine," *Journal of Sex & Marital Therapy* 29, no. 3 (2003): 207–13, doi: 10.1080/00926230390155104; and Andrea Ledda et al., "Investigation of a Complex Plant Extract for Mild to Moderate Erectile Dysfunction in a Randomized, Double-Blind, Placebo-Controlled, Parallel-Arm Study," *BJU International* 106, no. 7 (2010): 1030–33, doi: 10.1111/j.1464-410x.2010.09213.x.

16. Stanislavov and Nikolova, "Treatment of Erectile Dysfunction."

17. Takashi Suzuki et al., "The Effects on Plasma L-Arginine Levels of Combined Oral L-Citrulline and L-Arginine Supplementation in Healthy Males," *Bioscience, Biotechnology, and Biochemistry* 81, no. 2 (2016): 372–75, doi: 10.1080/09168451.2016.1230007.

18. Luigi Cormio et al., "Oral L-Citrulline Supplementation Improves Erection Hardness in Men with Mild Erectile Dysfunction," *Urology* 77, no. 1 (2011): 119–22, doi: 10.1016/j.urology.2010.08.028.

19. H. K. Choi, D. H. Seong, and K. H. Rha, "Clinical Efficacy of Korean Red Ginseng for Erectile Dysfunction," *International Journal of Impotence Research* 7, no. 3 (1995): 181–86.

20. Dai-Ja Jang et al., "Red Ginseng for Treating Erectile Dysfunction: A Systematic Review," *British Journal of Clinical Pharmacology* 66, no. 4 (2008): 444–50, doi: 10.1111/j.1365-2125.2008.03236.x.

21. Y. D. Choi et al., "Effects of Korean Ginseng Berry Extract on Sexual Function in Men with Erectile Dysfunction: A Multicenter, Placebo-Controlled, Double-Blind Clinical Study," *International Journal of Impotence Research* 25, no. 2 (2013): 45–50, doi: 10.1038 /ijir.2012.45.

22. Andreas Walther et al., "Psychobiological Protective Factors Modifying the Association between Age and Sexual Health in Men: Findings from the Men's Health 40+ Study," *American Journal of Men's Health* 11, no. 3 (2017): 737–47, doi: 10.1177/1557988316689238.

23. Paul J. Rizk et al., "Testosterone Therapy Improves Erectile Function and Libido in Hypogonadal Men," *Current Opinion in Urology* 27, no. 6 (2017): 511–15, doi: 10.1097/MOU.0000000000000442.

24. Edward David Kim and Stanley A. Brosman, "Erectile Dysfunction Treatment & Management: Approach Considerations, Pharmacologic Therapy, External Erection-Facilitating Devices," August 8, 2018, Medscape, https://emedicine.medscape.com /article/444220-treatment#d10.

25. Pamela I. Ellsworth, "Erectile Dysfunction (ED, Impotence)," MedicineNet, https://www.medicinenet.com/erectile_dysfunction _ed_impotence/article.htm#oral_phosphodiesterase_type_5 _pde5_inhibitors.

26. Otto I. Linet and Francis G. Ogrinc, "Efficacy and Safety of Intracavernosal Alprostadil in Men with Erectile Dysfunction," *New England Journal of Medicine* 334, no. 14 (1996): 873–77, doi: 10.1056/NEJM199604043341401.

27. Pamela I. Ellsworth, "Erectile Dysfunction (ED, Impotence)."

28. Lisette Hilton, "Shock Wave Therapy: ED Cure or Unproven Treatment?," *Urology Times*, August 6, 2019, https://www .urologytimes.com/mens-health/shock-wave-therapy-ed-cure -or-unproven-treatment.

29. "When Is Low-Intensity Shockwave Therapy a Good Option for Erectile Dysfunction?" Health Essentials from Cleveland Clinic, November 8, 2019, https://health.clevelandclinic.org/when-is

-low-intensity-shockwave-therapy-a-good-option-for-erectile
-dysfunction.

30. "Low-Intensity Shockwave Therapy," Health Essentials from
Cleveland Clinic.

31. Emma Alvarez Gibson, "Rev Up a Low Libido," WebMD, reviewed
December 13, 2015, https://www.webmd.com/men/features
/revving-up-low-libido; Melissa Conrad Stöppler, "Low Libido:
Symptoms & Signs," MedicineNet, https://www.medicinenet.
com/low_libido/symptoms.htm; "Medications That Affect Sexual
Dysfunction," Cleveland Clinic, reviewed October 25, 2016,
https://my.clevelandclinic.org/health/articles/9124-medications-
that-affect-sexual-function; and "Sex-Drive Killers: The Causes of
Low Libido," RxList, reviewed May 11, 2016, https://www.rxlist
.com/sex_drive_killers_slideshow/article.htm.

32. "Sexual Desire Disorder," *Psychology Today*.

33. John M. Grohol, "Hypoactive Sexual Desire Disorder Symptoms
(Males)," Psych Central, updated October 11, 2019, https://
psychcentral.com/disorders/hypoactive-sexual-desire
-disorder-symptoms.

34. Hnin Ei Thu et al., "*Eurycoma longifolia* as a Potential Adoptogen
of Male Sexual Health: A Systematic Review on Clinical Studies,"
Chinese Journal of Natural Medicines 15, no. 1 (2017): 71–80, doi:
10.1016/s1875-5364(17)30010-9.

35. Thu et al., "*Eurycoma longifolia* as a Potential Adoptogen of Male
Sexual Health."

36. Gustavo Francisco Gonzales et al., "Effect of *Lepidium meyenii*
(Maca), a Root with Aphrodisiac and Fertility-Enhancing Properties,
on Serum Reproductive Hormone Levels in Adult Healthy Men,"
Journal of Endocrinology 176, no. 1 (2003): 163–68, doi: 10.1677
/joe.0.1760163.

37. Rizk et al., "Testosterone Therapy Improves Erectile Function."

38. Carolyn A. Allan et al., "Testosterone Therapy Increases Sexual
Desire in Ageing Men with Low–Normal Testosterone Levels
and Symptoms of Androgen Deficiency," *International Journal of
Impotence Research* 20, no. 4 (2008): 396–401, doi: 10.1038
/ijir.2008.22.

Chapter 8: Supernutrition for the Prostate

1. Mahmoud ElJalby et al., "The Effect of Diet on BPH, LUTS and ED," *World Journal of Urology* 37, no. 6 (2018): 1001–5, doi: 10.1007 /s00345-018-2568-0.

2. Stacey A. Kenfield et al., "Mediterranean Diet and Prostate Cancer Risk and Mortality in the Health Professionals Follow-Up Study," *European Urology* 65, no. 5 (2014): 887–94, doi: 10.1016 /j.eururo.2013.08.009.

3. K. Das and N. Buchholz, "Benign Prostate Hyperplasia and Nutrition," *Clinical Nutrition ESPEN* 33 (2019): 5–11, doi: 10.1016 /j.clnesp.2019.07.015.

4. Yoon Jung Yang et al., "Comparison of Fatty Acid Profiles in the Serum of Patients with Prostate Cancer and Benign Prostatic Hyperplasia," *Clinical Biochemistry* 32, no. 6 (1999): 405–9, doi: 10.1016/s0009-9120(99)00036-3.

5. Katherine D. McManus, "A Practical Guide to the Mediterranean Diet," Harvard Health Blog, March 21, 2019, https://www.health .harvard.edu/blog/a-practical-guide-to-the-mediterranean-diet -2019032116194.

6. "WHO Calls on Countries to Reduce Sugars Intake among Adults and Children," World Health Organization, March 4, 2015, http:// www.who.int/mediacentre/news/releases/2015/sugar-guideline/en.

7. Ian F. Godsland, "Insulin Resistance and Hyperinsulinaemia in the Development and Progression of Cancer," *Clinical Science* 118, no. 5 (2009): 315–32, doi: 10.1042/CS20090399.

8. Chinedum Eleazu, Kate Eleazu, and Winner Kalu, "Management of Benign Prostatic Hyperplasia: Could Dietary Polyphenols Be an Alternative to Existing Therapies?" *Frontiers in Pharmacology* 8 (2017): 234, doi: 10.3389/fphar.2017.00234.

9. Eleazu, Eleazu, and Kalu, "Management of Benign Prostatic Hyperplasia."

10. Wendy Demark-Wahnefried et al., "Flaxseed Supplementation (Not Dietary Fat Restriction) Reduces Prostate Cancer Proliferation Rates in Men Presurgery," *Cancer Epidemiology Biomarkers & Prevention* 17, no. 12 (2008): 3577–87, doi: 10.1158/1055-9965.EPI-08-0008.

11. Wambui Grace Gathirua-Mwangi and Jianjun Zhang, "Dietary Factors and Risk of Advanced Prostate Cancer, *European Journal of Cancer Prevention* 23, no. 2 (2014): 96–109, doi: 10.1097 /cej.0b013e3283647394.

12. "Healthy Food Preparation: Reducing Toxicant Exposure," The Institute for Functional Medicine, https://www.ifm.org/news -insights/detox-food-and-toxins-safe-grilling-and-frying-methods.

13. Dyandra Parikesit et al., "The Impact of Obesity towards Prostate Diseases," *Prostate International* 4, no. 1 (2016): 1–6, doi: 10.1016 /j.prnil.2015.08.001.

14. "EWG's 2020 Shopper's Guide to Pesticides in Produce," Environmental Working Group, March 25, 2020, https://www.ewg .org/foodnews/summary.php.

15. Ilaria Paterni, Carlotta Granchi, and Filippo Minutolo, "Risks and Benefits Related to Alimentary Exposure to Xenoestrogens," *Critical Reviews in Food Science and Nutrition* 57, no. 16 (2017): 3384–404, doi: 10.1080/10408398.2015.1126547.

16. David W. Singleton and Sohaib A. Khan, "Xenoestrogen Exposure and Mechanisms of Endocrine Disruption," *Frontiers in Bioscience* 8, nos. 1–3 (2003): s110–18, doi: 10.2741/1010.

17. Gail S. Prins, "Endocrine Disruptors and Prostate Cancer Risk," *Endocrine-Related Cancer* 15, no. 3 (2008): 649–56, doi: 10.1677 /ERC-08-0043.

18. "2020 Shopper's Guide," Environmental Working Group.

19. Yelena B. Wetherill et al., "Xenoestrogen Action in Prostate Cancer: Pleiotropic Effects Dependent on Androgen Receptor Status," *Molecular Biology, Pathobiology and Genetics*, January 2005, https:// cancerres.aacrjournals.org/content/65/1/54.short.

20. Michelle N. Harvie and Tony Howell, "Could Intermittent Energy Restriction and Intermittent Fasting Reduce Rates of Cancer in Obese, Overweight, and Normal-Weight Subjects? A Summary of Evidence," *Advances in Nutrition: An International Review Journal* 7, no. 4 (2016): 690–705, doi: 10.3945/an.115.011767.

Chapter 9: Key Factors for Men's Health

1. W. Deng et al., "Telomerase Activity and Its Association with Psychological Stress, Mental Disorders, Lifestyle Factors and Interventions: A Systematic Review," *Psychoneuroendocrinology* 64 (2016): 150–63, doi: 10.1016/j.psyneuen.2015.11.017.

2. Terrence D. Hill et al., "Dimensions of Religious Involvement and Leukocyte Telomere Length," *Social Science & Medicine* 163 (2016): 168–75, doi: 10.1016/j.socscimed.2016.04.032.

3. Dean Ornish et al., "Increased Telomerase Activity and Comprehensive Lifestyle Changes: A Pilot Study," *The Lancet Oncology* 9, no. 11 (2008): 1048–57, doi: 10.1016 /S1470-2045(08)70234-1.

4. Mayo Clinic Staff, "Chronic Stress Puts Your Health at Risk," Mayo Clinic, https://www.mayoclinic.org/healthy-lifestyle/stress -management/in-depth/stress/art-20046037; and Markham Heid, "How Stress Affects Cancer Risk," MD Anderson Cancer Center, https://www.mdanderson.org/publications/focused-on-health /how-stress-affects-cancer-risk.h21-1589046.html.

5. Philip M. Ullrich, Susan K. Lutgendorf, and Karl J. Kreder, "Physiologic Reactivity to a Laboratory Stress Task among Men with Benign Prostatic Hyperplasia," *Urology* 70, no. 3 (2007): 487– 91, doi: 10.1016/j.urology.2007.04.048.

6. Michael Jan et al., "The Roles of Stress and Social Support in Prostate Cancer Mortality," *Scandinavian Journal of Urology* 50, no. 1 (2015): 47–55, doi: 10.3109/21681805.2015.1079796.

7. "Managing Stress," Cancer.Net, American Society of Clinical Oncology, July 2019, https://www.cancer.net/coping-with-cancer /managing-emotions/managing-stress.

8. Committee on Herbal Medicinal Products (HMPC), "Reflection Paper on the Adaptogenic Concept," European Medicines Agency, 2008, https://www.ema.europa.eu/en/documents/scientific -guideline/reflection-paper-adaptogenic-concept_en.pdf.

9. K. Chandrasekhar, Jyoti Kapoor, and Sridhar Anishetty, "A Prospective, Randomized Double-Blind, Placebo-Controlled Study of Safety and Efficacy of a High-Concentration Full-Spectrum Extract of Ashwagandha Root in Reducing Stress and Anxiety in Adults," *Indian Journal of Psychological Medicine* 34, no. 3 (2012): 255–62, doi: 10.4103/0253-7176.106022.

10. Biswajit Auddy et al., "A Standardized *Withania somnifera* Extract Significantly Reduces Stress-Related Parameters in Chronically Stressed Humans: A Double-Blind, Randomized, Placebo-Controlled Study," *Journal of the American Nutraceutical Association* 11, no. 1 (2008): 51–57.

11. Usharani Pingali, Raveendranadh Pilli, and Nishat Fatima, "Effect of Standardized Aqueous Extract of *Withania somnifera* on Tests of Cognitive and Psychomotor Performance in Healthy Human Participants," *Pharmacognosy Research* 6, no. 1 (2014): 12–18, doi: 10.4103/0974-8490.122912.

12. Mark Stengler, *The Natural Physician's Healing Therapies*, 2nd ed. reprint (New York: Penguin Group, 2010).

13. Yonghong Li et al., *"Rhodiola rosea L*.: An Herb with Anti-Stress, Anti-Aging, and Immunostimulating Properties for Cancer Chemoprevention," *Current Pharmacology Reports* 3, no. 6 (2017): 384–95, doi: 10.1007/s40495-017-0106-1.

14. Ion-George Anghelescu et al., "Stress Management and the Role of *Rhodiola rosea*: A Review," *International Journal of Psychiatry in Clinical Practice* 22, no. 4 (2018): 242–52, doi: 10.1080/13651501.2017.1417442.

15. Richard P. Brown, Patricia L. Gerbarg, and Zakir Ramazanov, "*Rhodiola rosea*: A Phytomedicinal Overview," *HerbalGram* 56 (2002): 40–52, http://cms.herbalgram.org/herbalgram/issue56/article2333.html.

16. Alan R. Gaby, *Nutritional Medicine* (Concord, NH: Fritz Perlberg, 2011).

17. Reidar Fossmark, Tom C. Martinsen, and Helge L. Waldum, "Adverse Effects of Proton Pump Inhibitors—Evidence and Plausibility," *International Journal of Molecular Sciences* 20, no. 20 (2019): 5203, doi: 10.3390/ijms20205203; and Joel J. Heidelbaugh, "Proton Pump Inhibitors and Risk of Vitamin and Mineral Deficiency: Evidence and Clinical Implications," *Therapeutic Advances in Drug Safety* 4, no. 3 (2013): 125–33, doi: 10.1177/2042098613482484.

18. Kristina Sauerwein, "Heartburn Drugs Linked to Fatal Heart and Kidney Disease, Stomach Cancer," Washington University School of Medicine in St. Louis, May 30, 2019, https://medicine.wustl.edu/news/popular-heartburn-drugs-linked-to-fatal-heart-disease-chronic-kidney-disease-stomach-cancer.

19. Suzanne H. Reuben, *Reducing Environmental Cancer Risk: What We Can Do Now*, President's Cancer Panel, April 2010, https://deainfo.nci.nih.gov/advisory/pcp/annualreports/pcp08-09rpt/pcp_report_08-09_508.pdf.

20. Audrey Blanc-Lapierre, Jean-François Sauvé, and Marie-Elise Parent, "Occupational Exposure to Benzene, Toluene, Xylene and Styrene and Risk of Prostate Cancer in a Population-Based Study," *Occupational & Environmental Medicine* 75, no. 8 (2018): 562–72, doi: 10.1136/oemed-2018-105058.

INDEX

Q

quercetin, 71–72
questionnaires
about BPH, 20
about LUTS, 47

R

race
BPH and, 16
prostate cancer and, 79
radiation therapy, 93
recipes
Anti-Inflammatory Carrot-Apple Juice, 181
Black Bean Soup with Cumin and Oregano, 184
Carrot-Miso Dressing, 190–191
Chunky Spiced Pear Sauce, 191
Creamy Tuna and Chickpea Spread, 190
Garlic Roasted Tofu with Cabbage and Onion, 185
Kale Chips, 189
Mango and Tahini Smoothie, 182
Moroccan Spiced Roasted Carrots, 188–189
Prostate Super Juice, 181
Salmon Cakes with Yogurt-Dill Sauce, 187–188
Turkey-Corn-Tomato Sauté, 186
Whole-Grain Banana-Blueberry Pancakes, 182–183
respiratory disease, 116, 143
Rhodiola rosea, 171
rye pollen extract
for BPH, 33–34
for CPPS, 69–71
for prostatitis, 12

S

Salmon Cakes with Yogurt-Dill Sauce (recipe), 187–188
sauna therapy, 174, 175
saw palmetto
for BPH, 34–37
for CPPS, 70–71
Sertoli cells, 117
serum total testosterone test, 123–124
sex drive. *see* libido
sex hormone–binding globulin (SHBG), 117–118, 123, 125
shock wave therapy, 149
sildenafil (Viagra), 145
sleep, testosterone deficiency and, 128
smoking
CPPS and, 66–67
ED and, 144
prostate cancer and, 79
smoothies
fiber in, 158
Mango and Tahini Smoothie (recipe), 182
polyphenols in, 157
somatic mutations, 80
sperm production and transport, 5–8
Standard American Diet (SAD), 127
Stanford University, 74
static prostate enlargement, 25
Stengler, Mark
Outside the Box Cancer Therapies, 104
Stengler Center for Integrative Medicine, 11
steroid abuse, 120
stress, 167–172
health role of, 167–168
herbal adaptogens for, 169–172
managing, 167, 168–169
prostate cancer and, 111
trauma and ED, 144
stress incontinence, 52
sugar, reducing consumption, 156

ACKNOWLEDGMENTS

My thanks to the team at Hay House for their concept of bringing a much-needed men's health and prostate book to market. Also to my wonderful wife, Angela, and my three kids: Mark Jr., Hope, and Luke. And most important, to the One we read about in the first sentence of Genesis, who created the incredible body design.

ABOUT THE AUTHOR

Dr. Mark Stengler is a naturopathic medical doctor who is in private practice in Encinitas, California. He is the best-selling author of more than 30 books, including *Prescription for Natural Cures* and *Outside the Box Cancer Therapies*. He has expertise in the field of integrative medicine, which combines the best of conventional and natural medicine. In 2019, Dr. Stengler was selected as the Top Doctor of the Year by the International Association of Top Professionals. He is also co-host of the syndicated radio show *Forever Young*. You can visit Dr. Stengler online at www.markstengler.com.

Hay House Titles of Related Interest

YOU CAN HEAL YOUR LIFE, the movie,
starring Louise Hay & Friends
(available as a 1-DVD program, an expanded 2-DVD set, and an
online streaming video)
Learn more at www.hayhouse.com/louise-movie

THE SHIFT, the movie,
starring Dr. Wayne W. Dyer
(available as a 1-DVD program, an expanded 2-DVD set, and an
online streaming video)
Learn more at www.hayhouse.com/the-shift-movie

***

*Cancer-Free with Food: A Step-by-Step Plan with 100+ Recipes to
Fight Disease, Nourish Your Body & Restore Your Health,* by Liana
Werner-Gray

Chris Beat Cancer: A Comprehensive Plan for Healing Naturally, by
Chris Wark

Mind Over Medicine: Scientific Proof That You Can Heal Yourself, by
Lissa Rankin, M.D.

*Radical Hope: 10 Key Healing Factors from Exceptional Survivors of
Cancer & Other Diseases,* by Kelly A. Turner, Ph.D., with Tracy
White

*The Truth about Cancer: What You Need to Know about Cancer's
History, Treatment, and Prevention,* by Ty M. Bollinger

All of the above are available at your local bookstore,
or may be ordered by contacting Hay House (see next page).

***

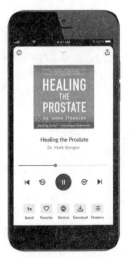